Feeling Great!

Feeling

Enhancing

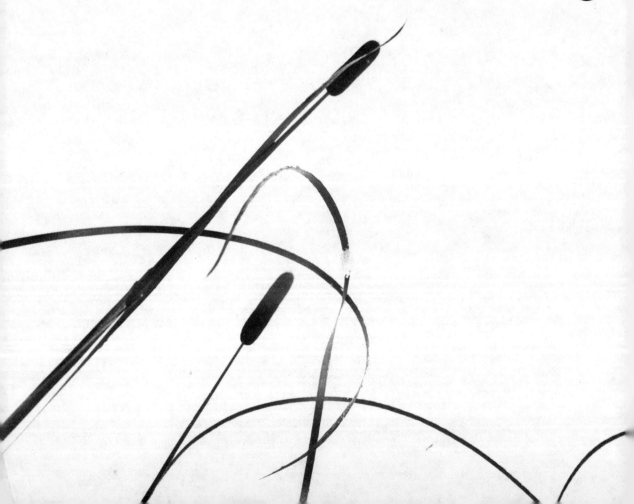

Great!

Your Health & Well-Being

by Jeanne Segal, Ph.D.

Photographs by Lynne Ericksson

1983
NEWCASTLE PUBLISHING CO., INC.
NORTH HOLLYWOOD, CALIFORNIA

Second Printing, 1983

Published by Newcastle Publishing Co., Inc.,
        P.O. Box 7589, Van Nuys, CA 91409

ISBN 0-87877-069-0

Cover design by Riley K. Smith
Book design by Craig Caughlan
Typeset by Jonathan Peck

PRINTED IN THE UNITED STATES OF AMERICA
9 8 7 6 5 4 3 2

I gratefully acknowledge the perspective and skills taught me by Jean Houston, Harold Stone, William Brugh Joy, Margaret Paul and Robert Segal; the opportunities afforded me by the Center for the Healing Arts, and International College; and last, but not least, the consistent loving support of my family and friends.

Table of Contents

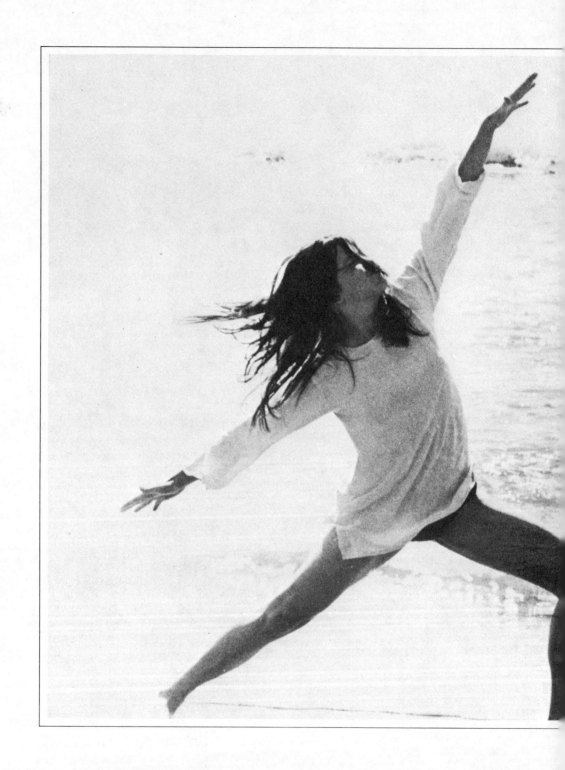

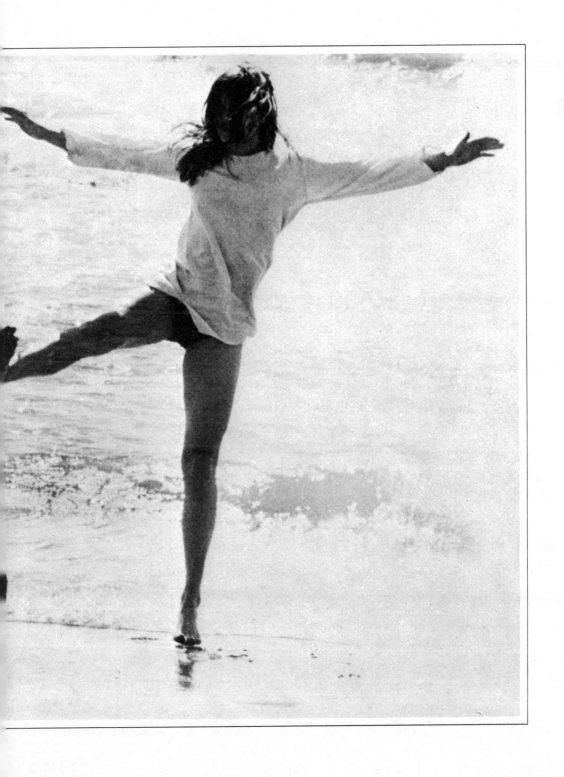

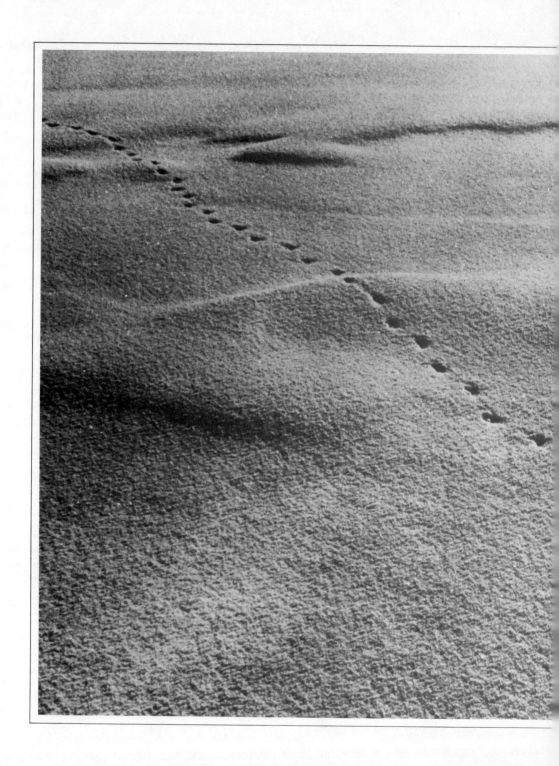

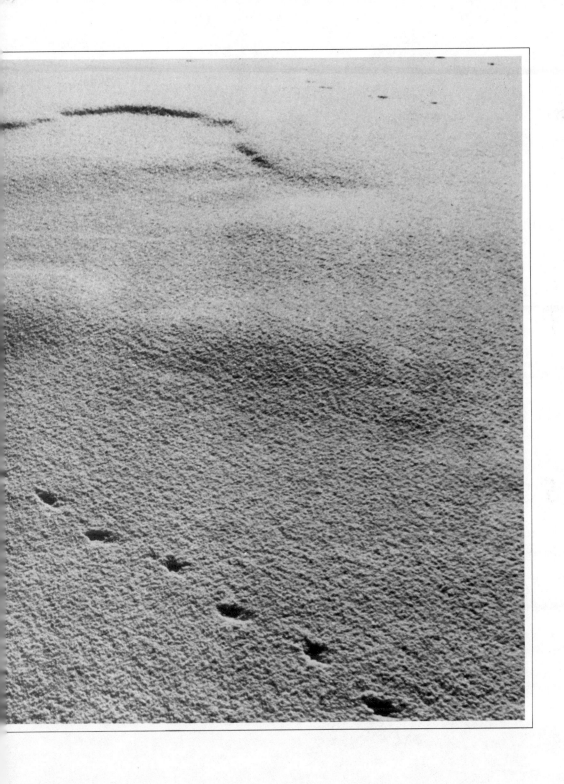

Foreword

In the last minutes of the eleventh hour there arise the Ones Who Call Us To Remember Who We Really Are. Out in front or working quietly behind the scenes, in shrill or in gentle tones, they remind us that we are at that point at the great divide where we have no choice but to grow or die. They present us with awesome challenge, telling us the human race has evolved to have a remarkably fine psycho-social instrument, but that now we must use, create, work and deepen with this instrument in ways that hitherto have remained more mythic than real.

The convergence of cross-cultural styles and of ancient wisdom with modern technology, of quantum physics with mystic union — these are the seedings and quickenings that prove that the Zeit is getting very geisty and that the opportunity has never been greater for the possible human to emerge among great numbers of humankind.

In clear and conversational tones Jeanne Segal has written a guidebook to human possibilities and the recovery of the dimensions of ourselves. Drawing upon her many years of study and application of methods in human potentiation, she has assembled some of the most valuable and practical of these techniques and managed to present them in a style at once charming and easy to follow. The readers would be warned, however, that in following the procedures she outlines, there is the likelihood that they will find themselves in the midst of an evolutionary adventure story. They may enter upon the path of a futuristic Everyman questing beyond the constraints of present human sensibilities to a place of unfolding, which, once it begins, can never really be stopped.

Again, be warned about this book. Behind its guileless guise is an evolutionary time bomb. But then that is to be expected, for Jeanne Segal is surely a member of the Ones Who Call Us To Remember Who We Really Are.

JEAN HOUSTON
The Foundation for Mind Research
Pomona, New York 10970

March, 1980

Preface

This book gives me the opportunity to touch people with ideas, inspirations, and concerns I care deeply about.

My intention has been to create a bridge between esoteric language and practices of what has been termed the "New Age" and the language, needs and interests of people from other walks of life. So often, verbal communication is a barrier between people rather than a road of access. This book is an attempt to go beyond the limits of language to a source of common experience.

Finally, to my great delight, I have had the opportunity to synthesize and utilize many experiences, including some that were unpleasant, while working on this book. All that has happened to me has revealed new meanings and purposes once again, and I continue my search for greater understanding, deeper awareness and fuller sharing of all that I have come across in my own journey toward well-being.

Prelude:
The Holistic Journey

Once upon a time, there lived a king and queen who awaited with anticipation the birth of a child. When the child was born, a powerful and beneficent magician gave it a crown made of a precious and marvelous metal that was capable of magically expanding so that the crown might be placed on the child's head forever. There were other miraculous properties alluded to at the time, but not revealed. Now, around the four sides of this wonderful crown were very tiny holes, almost imperceptibly small, but as the child grew, the crown grew and the holes in it enlarged until much of its original harmony was lost, as the crown now contained four large gaping holes. This was a source of disturbance, because the crown, having remained permanently affixed to the head, was an integral part of the now young adult, and, to tell the truth, it really didn't look good any more! The magician was called for and the king asked, "Why did you present our child with a crown that has lost its beauty?" The magician answered that the crown needed only to be set on each of its sides with precious stones in order to make it harmonious and beautiful. The magician then took the youthful heir into his chamber and spoke of four interconnected roads that contained in their dust the precious stones that would complete the crown. Because these roads were continuously intersected by others that led nowhere, the magician gave the heir apparent, of all things—a roach! Now the roach was not a particularly attractive traveling companion and at first the young heir objected. But the magician insisted, pointing out that the roach is loyal, dependable and has a very keen sense of smell. The heir relented, and with the roach set off to journey the four roads in quest of the precious stones.

Years passed in the pursuit of the first stone. The first road was very steep and rocky. Thick brush all but covered it, and, as the magician predicted, there were many side roads indistinguishable from the main one. Real physical strength was required to hike this steep path. The heir was exhausted at first and had to stop frequently for breath. Gradually, however, the heir's body strengthened and eventually the steep and rocky crevices were traversed with grace and ease. At about this time the roach bumped into the first stone, a ruby lying in a pile of dust on the road. At first it appeared to have little luster, but the heir, thinking to wash it with a little drinking water, then polished it with a bit of blouse. To the heir's amazement this cleansing process revealed a stone of extraordinary color and brilliance.

The second path began where the first ended and was equally grueling, for it not only twisted and turned, but also undulated constantly such that balance was impossible to maintain and the traveler was troubled by nausea. The heir became uncertain and childlike. Had resolve been shallow, or the roach a less steady companion, the heir might have turned back many times over the years this difficult course was traveled. Eventually, however, the second stone, a golden topaz, was discovered like the first, lying in the road. This too required washing and polishing before its profound beauty revealed itself.

As before, the third road began where the second had ended, and this one was truly a puzzlement, for the forward way was blocked continuously with barriers every few feet, such that it was necessary to move to the left or right, and sometimes completely around as in a maze. In order to traverse this confusing path, the heir's mind needed sharpening. Anything less than the clearest and most circumspect of thinking led to walking in circles. In this situation the heir came to value still more the slower, more cautious pace of the roach and found it to produce in the end the most dependable progress.

Again, many years passed until the third precious stone, a purple-blue chunk of lapis lazuli, was discovered, lying in the dust of the road. This too required washing and polishing. Now three great stones were secure in the crown of the heir apparent who was, by now, not so young and somewhat weary. The final path lay ahead, yet out of view, for a silver mist covered the countryside at the point where the third road ended and the fourth began.

Because of the weariness and because little could be seen anyway, this path was traveled with eyes closed, surrendering the lead completely to the roach who sniffed through the mist. Traveling this way opened a whole new world of awareness. The heir experienced the breeze, the sun, the dust in the road, the trees and bushes as indistinguishable from the hands, the feet, the cheek that touched them. Again, many years passed, and by this time a life of searching had grown satisfying and no pressure was felt to secure anything. Nonetheless, the fourth and final stone was also found. When the dust was washed away, a crystal appeared of such shape, clarity and depth that it illuminated the universe. This final stone the aged and trembling hand placed in the fourth opening, and, at that very moment, the crown's truly miraculous nature was fully revealed, for the heir became in an instant youthful—standing once more erect under the great crown now brilliant and balanced with the addition of the four precious stones.

With wondering eyes, the heir turned to thank the faithful roach and beheld in its stead a magnificent and strangely exciting figure. Hand in hand the two turned toward a clearing that contained a dazzling palace, the doors of which opened to welcome them.

A great celebration marked this event, and all who dwelt in the palace and lands surrounding as far as the eye could see celebrated the "well-being" of all.

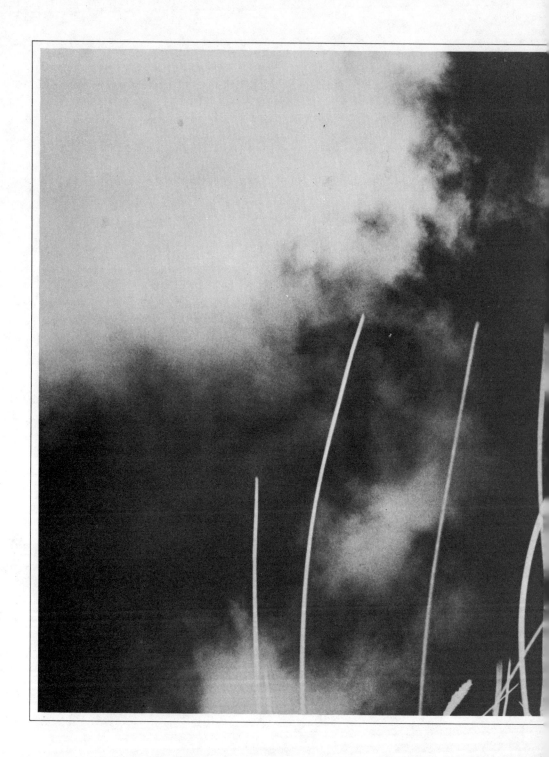

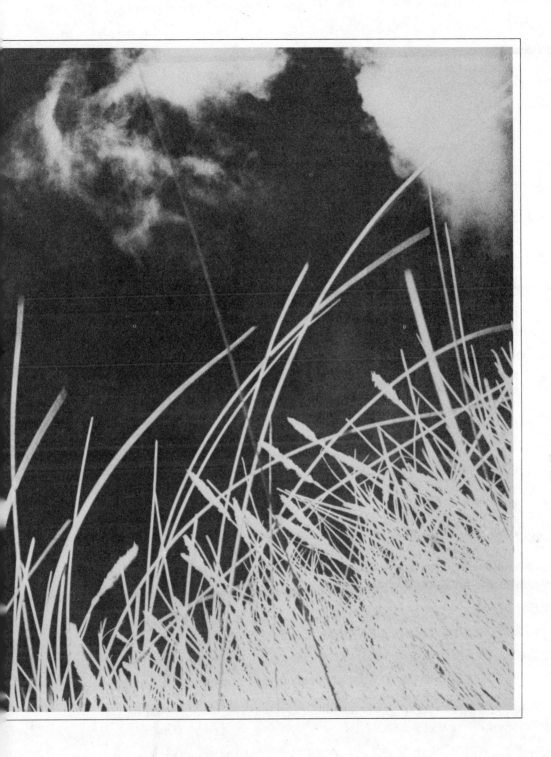

1

The Pursuit Of Wonder-Fullness

You have a right to enthusiastic well-being. You're programmed for it. *You have a tremendous genetic endowment of which only a small fraction is used.* It's there for a purpose and that purpose is to be fully alive! This book is for those who are ready and willing to feel "wonder-full." By this I mean relaxed, vital, soft, secure and full of the wonder and joy that comes with connection to the universe.

When I suggest the possibility of life lived within the contest of wonder and enthusiasm to clients and students,[1] they often respond with disbelief. "Who, me? I'm not gifted, or a mystic." "Is it really possible for an average person like myself to feel 'that way' while taking care of a home and pursuing material well-being?" The answer is yes, if that's what you want.

Many of us grew up in environments that erased or severely limited our sense of possibility.[2] Intense joy and experiences of wonder, assuming they ever existed in the first place, ended with childhood, as did growth and unfolding. If this is your belief, acknowledge it, along with any others that limit your sense of possibility; but acknowledge at the same time that just as you were taught, and learned, to see yourself and life as limited, so you can also be taught, and learn, to lift the restrictions and open to new possibilities for a healthier, fuller, richer, more joyous and extended life.

How to use this book

I suggest that in addition to reading, you "experience" this book through its exercises. Doing the exercises—which I also call "experiences"— will teach you what you know about yourself, and that is what will extend your life!

24

The exercises that have to do with visualization have purposely been written in skeletal form. This enables you to embellish each with sights sounds, smells, touch, tastes and inspirations that make them personally pleasurable for you. One person's imagined glorious field of flowers can be another's hay fever! Don't be afraid to add words or whole scenes if this intensifies the experience for you—and it probably will. *Some people prefer to engage in new experiences by themselves while others get more out of sharing them.* If you're one of those individuals who is apt to get more out of something when accompanied by another, engage a loved one, a friend or acquaintance, several perhaps, in exploring the ideas and processes described in this book. While this book starts with yourself and where you are, it can be used by an entire family to deepen and enrich the lives of all.

Most of the visual experiences contained in the text are brief and simple enough to be easily committed to memory. You may, however, wish to use a tape recorder if one is handy, because it is simpler and easier to relax and concentrate without the pressure of having to recall instructions. The same holds true, of course, if someone is available to read you the instructions.

The material in *Feeling Great* draws from the work of Jean Houston, Ph.D., Harold Stone, Ph.D., Brugh Joy, M.D., Margret and Jorden Paul and my own research and development. In order to acknowledge the significant contributions made by others, and to describe the research process, notes are included at the end of each chapter. In addition, the Bibliography located at the end of the book includes the sources that inspired much of the material and some of the exercises outlined in the book. Turn to this list of books if you want to go further—or deeper.

Be aware that *none of the processes described in this book require the investment of a great deal of time.* In fact, if you were to turn over a small fraction of the minutes you spend ruminating about past or future events and devote them instead to the processes suggested in this book, you would have all the time you need.

Those experiences that you find particularly meaningful will become even more so if you give them a moment's attention every day for three or four weeks. Five or ten minutes may be time enough to invest in recalling the experience and its meaning. In so doing you will have it easily available to memory. For years I have instructed clients to tape their sessions and replay the tapes, by themselves, within thirty-six hours. In so doing, people learn in a fraction of the time it usually takes. Years ago I chanced on this technique when I was a student nearly failing a required statistics class. Later a teacher told me that repetition within a relatively short time frame affects the brain in a way we associate with new learning.

This book and the experiences contained within it together afford you the opportunity to expand your awareness of yourself and your relationship with the universe.[3] Moreover, transformation, the process of integrating this awareness, can take place within the context of a contemporary life that is practically and materially focused. All that is required is intention. In moving from intentionality to practice, begin by visualizing the intention. See yourself vividly doing that which you intend. Hear, smell, touch, taste the experience. In so doing, your mind has begun the process. You don't actually have to visually see your intended activity, provided you hear, smell, touch or taste it vividly.

If it is indeed your intention to broaden your awareness, to explore new possibilities for enjoying greater physical, mental, emotional and spiritual "well-being," you will find that the time and the energy to read this book comes easier. It may mean getting up earlier and/or going to bed later, but you'll do it. You may complete this workbook in a few weeks or it may take you many years. It really doesn't matter. Each person has his or her own rhythm and pace. If yours is slower, honor it. You will learn and experience more following a course that is natural for you than forcing yourself to be like someone else.

When you're in a process of working toward becoming all that you can be mentally, physically, emotionally and spiritually, you begin a journey that leads increasingly to joy, well-being and "wonder-fullness."

Bon Voyage!

Notes to Chapter I

[1] All of the material in this workbook has been used successfully over a period of five years in private classes, classes at Everywoman's Village and groups at the Center for the Healing Arts, a holistic health center. My students included individuals ranging in age from fifteen to seventy-eight and in all stages of health and well-being.

[2] As a practicing psychotherapist for many years, I have discussed early life impressions with hundreds of people.

[3] I have led transformational groups for very successful business and professional people, as well as students and young mothers. All found the time to engage in the processes and exercises described in this book.

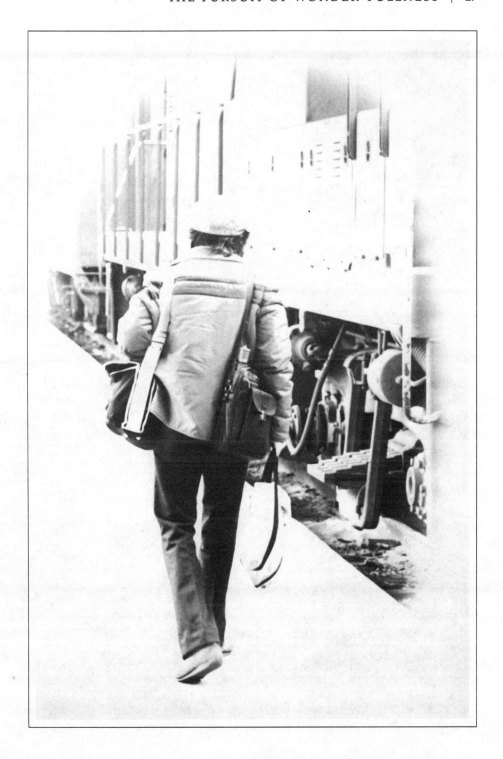

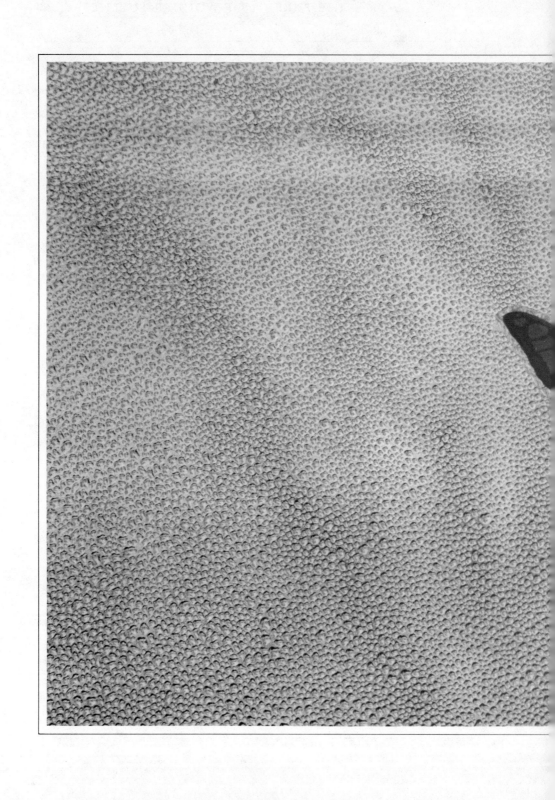

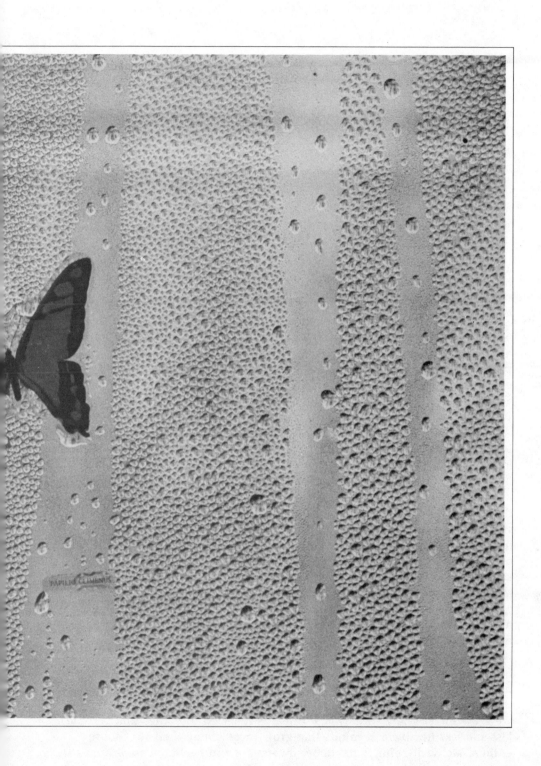

PAPILIO CLIMENUS

2

Beginning with Awareness

Awareness is the key to extending and enhancing your life. The more we become aware of, the more we can appreciate and enjoy. I get a great deal more out of the experience of watching a football game when I perceive the complexity of the plays. If I have played football, then my experience, as a viewer, is not only mental, but also physical and emotional. The viewing process is no longer passive, but rather active. Participation in any of life's events is enlivened and enriched by increased awareness. Awareness also increases the possible choices we have. For example, if I feel like eating and I'm aware that the feeling has more to do with loneliness than hunger I may call up a friend rather than eat.

One way of becoming increasingly aware is to collect more and more information. This can be a tedious and time-consuming process. Another way is to extend perception so that all of our experiences are richer, juicier, more engaging and fully satisfying. Moreover this process of stretching awareness or consciousness doesn't require our committing a great deal of time to it. Many of the experiences in this book can be done standing or waiting in line, driving or at odd moments of the day when chances are you would be daydreaming anyway.

In addition to stretching your capacity to appreciate life and bringing about choice, enhanced awareness is much more likely to produce a state of optimum physical health than that of limited awareness. Experience working with seriously ill people has taught me that *a good reason for dying is not knowing how to live fully! Life is a process and if we are not in the process of living, we are in the process of dying.* When we hold on to our customary patterns, avoiding that which is challenging and unknown, we grow increasingly stiff. This stiffness is reflected in bodies that become less and less flexible and minds that grow increasingly tired. To choose enthusiastic well-being is to choose awareness and health.

Freeze!

Begin where you are this instant. Exactly how do you feel . . . can you tell me? What criteria do you use? Can you check your body, your stomach or chest for gut reactions, or do you ask your mind to answer the following question, "How am I doing?" Go ahead—check it out. If you haven't already done so, observe exactly how you feel this instant, and hold onto an awareness of the feeling for a few seconds.

Did you surprise yourself at all? *Most of the time people don't really pay careful attention to exactly how they're feeling,* unless of course their feeling is very bad. In fact, many define feeling good as the absence of bad feeling. How about you? If you are typical, this appraisal won't be a particularly easy thing to do. There are a number of good reasons why self-observation is difficult. In the first place, unless you are the introspective type, self-observation may simply be a habit that you are not acquainted with. You may have been trained to be a careful observer of others or of things but not necessarily of yourself.

Another good reason for not paying close attention to what we feel is that we don't like what we find when we stop to notice. We judge our feelings to be bad or wrong. Perhaps we've overeaten—we feel overly full and criticize ourselves for lacking self-control; or we feel envious and criticize ourselves for being petty; or we feel bored and criticize ourselves for not having the initiative to find something interesting to do . . . and so it goes! *When self-observation is paired with self-criticism and judgment, of course we avoid it!*

When we have the desire to do things in a new way, insufficient self-awareness is an obstacle. New ongoing patterns and behaviors rarely result from the simple intent to do things differently. How many times have you made up your mind to stop something or to start something, which for a short time you are able to do? However, just at the point where you think you licked the old pattern or behavior there you are doing it again! This happens to all of us again and again and it's the result of beginning without sufficient understanding and acceptance of our current behaviors. We always do what we do for good reasons, although these reasons may be quite obscure to us. What happens is that we go along changing for the good reasons we consciously have until we encounter the equally good reasons we have for the way we've been doing it all along. The place therefore to begin is with a very careful and nonjudgmental look at exactly what we are doing!

There are a number of ways to begin collecting information about yourself and the experiences that follow will give you an opportunity to try some of these, but before you begin the process, you'll need to create for yourself an impartial, exacting observer.[1] Pretend that you're a reporter from Mars collecting information about the behaviors, feelings, and thoughts of an earthling—you! Now as a reporter from Mars, you not only observe all external activity but have knowledge of internal activity as well. It all interests you, and since you have no human judgments, everything you see is exactly as it should be. Feeling bored, angry or lonely isn't bad—it's just a feeling to take note of in the context of what the earthling is doing, as are feelings of well-being and joy. One more thing about this reporter from Mars: he or she has a sense of humor so that even though the job of reporting takes concentration and dedication, it's fun too. With the objectivity of a reporter from Mars, you are now prepared to begin a process that holds the key for unlocking countless doors in an attempt to recognize old patterns and create new ones.

The following exercise will develop in you a capacity for impartial self-observation.

Exercise 1—Creating a Witness to Yourself

1. Begin by getting yourself a notebook in which you can jot down observations. I prefer a chart form myself, with two columns—one with the heading, "What Am I Doing?" and the other with the heading, "How Do I Feel?"

2. Ask yourself, "What am I doing?" Note all that you're involved in. Presumably you're reading this particular passage; what else are you doing—watching TV, daydreaming or listening to the neighbors fight?

3. Ask your body how you feel doing whatever it is that you're doing.

   a. Generally, your mind will tell you *what* you're doing and your body will tell you *how* you feel doing it. So if you are not used to paying attention to how you feel, concentrate on the different parts of your body: feet, calves, knees, thighs, pelvis, stomach, chest, shoulders, back, back of neck, hands, arms, face and head.

   If you're having trouble identifying sensations in different parts of your body, try tensing or squeezing each part for ten seconds. As you release the tension, observe the feeling that comes with the release and hold onto it for a few seconds.

   b. Another method for enhancing awareness of body parts is to lie on your back on the floor, palms down, to music with the volume turned up. Pretend the music is playing *you* or entering and moving through the various parts of your body—retain the sensation for a few seconds after the music ends.

4. Assess the information that you have collected. Now give every-thing that you're aware of a general rating of *NOT OK, OK* or *VERY GOOD*. Perhaps imagining a scale from −5 to +5 with zero in the middle will make it easier for you to do this. Remember that no score or rating is "bad"−you're simple gathering information about yourself. Hold this awareness for a few seconds.

    a. If you're having trouble concentrating or identifying feelings, note this objectively and estimate your overall self-awareness with whatever information you are able to collect.

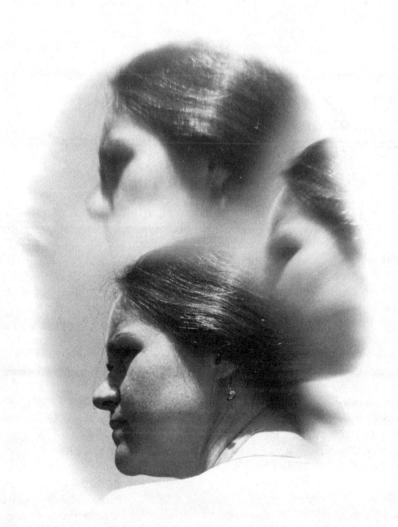

5. Resolve to try out this assessment during waking hours every two or three hours for at least three consecutive days. In this way you are building an inner clock that brings you the gift of self-awareness quickly in small doses that will increase with time. After a few weeks or a few months, if you so intend, your clock may go off more often, bringing information every hour or every twenty minutes until you have developed the state of awareness that I call "the witness"[2] In the witness state, you will find yourself aware of what you're doing and how you feel doing it *much of the time.*

With this skill under your belt, you will have access not only to more subtle emotions and fresh sensations in your body, but also to a process of tapping into your pool of intuitive and creative intelligence.

What do you do when you become aware of feelings you never felt before and the experience is upsetting?

It isn't unusual for people who seriously begin to track their feeling and energy patterns to discover things about themselves that they didn't expect and don't like. For example, a soft-spoken, sweet-mannered young woman about two weeks into class said shakenly, "I'm angry *all* the time and that scares me: especially for my helpless children." Of course, there is nothing particularly pleasant about discovering that you spend most or even a significant part of your life experiencing anger, or hurt, or fear, etc. . . . but the truth is that whatever you discover has been there all along anyway and without awareness most likely will remain so.

Moreover, *there is real danger attached to ignoring awareness of difficult or unpleasant emotions.* Sooner or later feelings make themselves known, and ignored feelings are apt to surface uncontrollably in indirect and inappropriate ways with ourselves and with others. For example, stress provoked by unrecognized anger or fear can lead to physical or emotional illness. The grinding of teeth during the night, hemorrhoids, ulcers, emotional depression and sometimes much more serious physical and mental disease forms can be expressions of feelings disowned by conscious awareness. Our relationships with other people can also be affected by emotions that increase stress in ways of which we have little or no awareness. Others may find it unpleasant to be around us or we may experience ourselves uncontrollably saying and doing things that we know are inappropriate or unwise, such as withdrawing from people and situations we care about, or venting our anger on an innocent person.

To bring something to awareness is to begin to have choices about what you will do with it. Anger consciously experienced as feeling or emotion can also be perceived by the mind as a certain kind of energy—a force that can be put behind an intention for physical activity or creative expression. You can, for example, run or engage in other forms of physical activity using your anger or righteous indignation as you would make use of wind behind a sail—a force that pushes you past inertia and lethargy to the form your intention takes. Angry people can be highly productive when they move that energy out into the world in a constructive way. The key lies in the capacity to be constructive with the energy. Think of it as fuel. Visualize it as an empowering force—energy that can be harnessed behind creative new projects and ways of being.

Hurt and pain also have appropriate as well as inappropriate forms. Be they emotional or physical, they can be perceived as teachers—as an indication that we are not doing something we need to do for ourselves or a statement that we are engaged in a process or processes that we ought to forego. Pain and hurt viewed in this context are not punishment or retribution, but opportunities to become aware of that which you were not aware of before, and thereby opportunities to ultimately extend well-being and the quality of life.

A note about writing things down

If you don't want to take a large notebook with you wherever you go, a pocket-size one will do. The point is that some type of written notation is important initially.[3] What you're doing is setting up a pattern that reminds you to pay close attention to yourself, and writing reinforces this new habit that you are building. People will tell me that they do not have to write things down in order to remember and pay careful attention to them—they can recall what they did and how they felt. The only people I really accept this statement from are those who can consistently recall their dreams intact without writing *them* down! If you can do this without taking written notes, you probably don't need to write these observations down either; otherwise, do it even though it may seem tedious the first few times.

Continue to build and polish your self-awareness until you can objectively, at any time, move away from yourself for an instant to observe what you're doing and feeling.

The place of energy in our intent to create new patterns and ways of being

A basic and essential part of any creative new system is energy. It takes some energy to set about doing almost anything and it takes a considerable amount to begin to do things differently. That's why beginning a new project at the end of the day (or the beginning of the day if you're a night person) is usually a bust! It's much easier to begin and keep going when you start during that time of day when you normally feel the most energized.

Most of us first become aware of energy as a sensation of liveliness, excitement or well-being contained within our physical bodies. It's very apparent, for example, when you have just completed an invigorating run or swim, or the minute you receive very good news, that you feel uplifted. Listening to your favorite piece of music can do the same thing for you as can being with someone you love very much. It's as if everything becomes clearer, lighter — there is more joy to life. Energy is also defined by some as get up and go or enthusiasm. It is all these and much, much more.

Your immediate need for becoming familiar with subtler forms of energy is that in order to explore the new possibilities and experiences contained in this book, you will need to draw on all the energy you can lay claim to, both internally and externally, and perhaps releasing dormant energy in yourself. If you are going to do this, you will need to awaken to the concept that *all we experience as reality has energetic quality as well as material quality.* Albert Einstein proved that all matter can be converted into energy, and the new physics is demonstrating that everything has an energy component that our own energy interacts with and is affected by.[4] To begin to perceive yourself, what you do, other people, events and things in terms of their energy as well as their material form is to begin to open your consciousness to a vast new realm of possibilities that illuminate and support well-being.

Moreover, to the extent that you are becoming an objective self-observer, you have already begun sensing less apparent feelings and experiences. You have entered into the process of observing subtler energy forms.

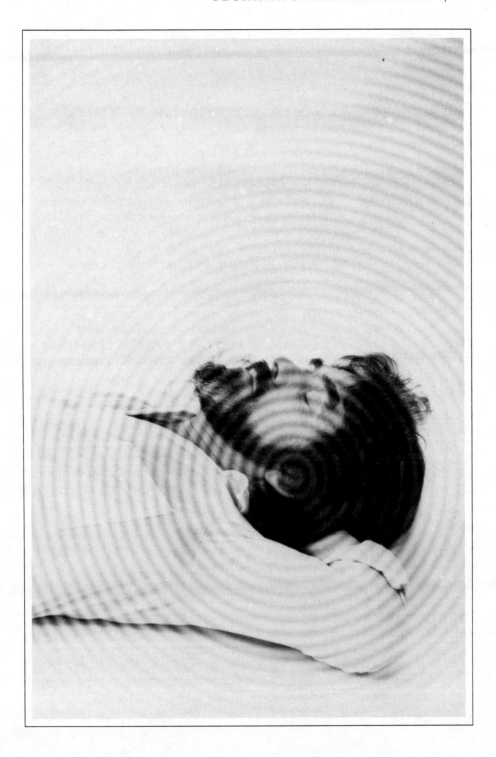

The following exercise will develop your capacity to recognize the effects of various energies on your inner awareness of well-being.

Exercise 2 — Creating a Personal Energy Scanner

1. Imagine that your time clock has turned into a radar-like energy scanner, which periodically, during the day, appraises what you are doing, how you feel doing it and the environment — all at an energy level. The scanner will stop and take into account your sense of feeling uplifted or brought down by a situation, person or event. For example, you just had lunch with your best friend. Do you feel uplifted or deflated by the experience? Take another situation — a family gathering — what's your awareness now? Did the scanner register a plus or minus in terms of the energy generated by the experience? Chances are that if you pay careful attention, you will experience energy shifts as you move from situation to situation during the day.

2. Write your observations down as notations or in chart form with the following headings: "What Am I Doing?" — "How Do I Feel Doing What I'm Doing?" — "How Is My Energy Being Affected?" Continue to make notations until the process requires no effort on your part to make the observations. In other words, continue until this process is habitual.

3. Stay in the "witness state." Remember that the ease with which you will be able to tune into the energetic quality of people and experiences is determined by the objectivity of your scanning device. A decrease of energy is not necessarily bad or good — it's just something to take notice of in the context of your conscious intentions. You will begin to observe much more in terms of how your energy lifts or diminishes if you maintain a neutral but interested posture.

It becomes at times humorous to observe our behaviors in light of our conscious objectives. For example, watching TV is sure to put me soundly to sleep no matter how energetic I feel when I turn it on. Yet I can't tell you how many times I said to myself that I was going to watch TV for an hour and then pay bills or write letters or whatever — activities that require a measure of alertness on my part. It would make a lot more sense from the standpoint of my energy level to watch TV on evenings when I want only to sleep! As you become aware of yourself in terms of energy you begin to be increasingly in charge of your life — that is, behavior more and more lines up with and supports conscious intentions, and that which you think you want, you begin to get.

In addition to experiencing energy contained within your body you can also learn to experience the energy that lies outside of your physical body, the energy field that surrounds it, and that of others. I've already mentioned the feeling of being lifted or depressed. This feeling can be also validated by other ways of observing energy. Today, for example, there are sensing devices such as Kirlian photographic equipment that pick up energetic emanations, but your mind/brain system is as capable as these machines of doing this, and with practice you can begin to sense the same thing directly.

You may also train yourself to recognize energy. When people see auras, what they're observing is the energy emanating from the body. In the section on expanding awareness of your mind/brain system, I will introduce you to experiences that facilitate developing the skill of sensing energy. The thing to keep in mind at this point is that it is a skill which, like any other, can be learned through effort and patience.[5]

The following exercise will help you to pay careful attention to energy as you experience it right now in relation to people and events outside of yourself.

Exercise 3 — Gaining Awareness of Energy That Surrounds You

1. Plan to spend three to ten days observing yourself, your activities, the people and events you come into contact with in terms of energy input or outgo. Take notes on or chart these events.

2. Ask yourself the following questions as you continue to observe. "How enlivened or depleted do I feel as I move from situation to situation or person to person during the day?" For example, you may notice as you scan or appraise your energy level that while an hour ago you felt exhausted and unable to move, you've started to do something you enjoy or see someone you like and now feel awake, alert and very interested in what you're doing.

3. Track your observations carefully, taking notice of the feelings contained within your physical body as you make this assessment.

4. Keep this up until you find yourself making these kinds of observations automatically.

Moving back into your role as the objective reporter from Mars will facilitate your gathering this information, and remember — take a sense of humor with you. If you can't smile a little at yourself, then you probably can't even see yourself — enjoy!

Gaining awareness of your thought patterns

Now at this point you are hopefully paying more and more attention to that which you do and that which you feel. You are becoming an objective observer of yourself, and perhaps of others too. You check your energy level, and the relative pleasure or dis-ease that accompanies your activities and the situations you find yourself in. You are probably noticing that there are discernible patterns in your life—certain activities, certain people that predictably elicit a type of feeling. Some of these are positive, others are negative. I suggest that you pay particular attention to the positive impressions with the intention of experiencing these more often.

To this process of noting relationships between doing and feeling or sensing I am now going to suggest an additional consideration: What is it that you think about and how does that affect what you feel?

What percentage of the time do you spend daydreaming? Fifty to seventy-five percent[6] is the average according to studies on college students. We all spend a great deal of time in our heads thinking about what could happen or what we wish would happen, or what we're afraid might happen or what happened that we wish hadn't, etc. In other words, we spend a considerable amount of time picturing life inside our heads.

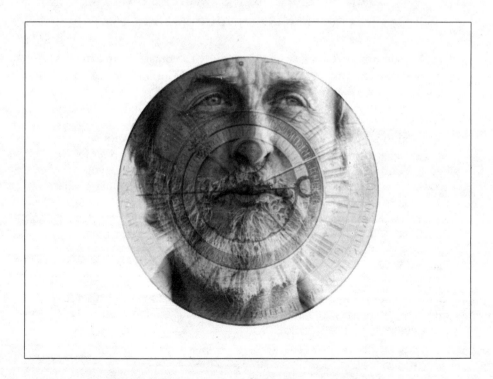

The following exercise will help you to become aware of your thought patterns.

Exercise 4 — Watching the Picture Show Inside Your Head

1. Decide to begin paying careful, objective attention to your day-time mind pictures.

2. Ask yourself the following questions: What are the scenarios that I create — the discussions, the situations, the people I love and hate, win and lose within my mind's eye?

3. View these pictures and plots as if you were watching a series of short-subject films during the day.

4. Do this for a week.

Note-taking will quicken your awareness as will sharing these stories out loud with a friend. Again, remember to remind yourself to withhold judgment of that which you experience. Our fantasies consciously witnessed can be terribly embarrassing or even downright frightening. The best part about sharing them out loud is that you soon find out you're not as peculiar as you thought you were. "Me, too" is the response people get time and again after sharing embarrassing fantasies.

Keep in mind that "seeing" does not necessarily necessitate a visual experience. You may sense or hear rather than "see" with your mind's eye. If you have been watching yourself imagining for a week and taking notes, you can begin to start perceiving patterns — themes that recur. Ask yourself what scripts are replayed and what feelings are generated by these imaginings — particularly the ones you rerun again and again. Note the correlation between the thought process and the feeling. Perhaps you have started to notice that you can be in a bad mood and turn it into a good mood with a particular fantasy or the reverse. You're really feeling OK or even good and you put on an old scenario that fills you with anger or resentment. Many people do this all the time, not realizing to what extent they are consciously choosing to feel a particular way simply by selecting certain thought patterns. Watch yourself affecting how you feel with what you think, and continue to write down your observations. This is an exercise that can be practiced profitably for a lifetime!

There is another aspect of this process that's intriguing. Fantasy suggests that which we really want and need, although, like the night dream, the message may be somewhat obscure. For example, recurring sexual fantasies that focus more on changing partners and settings than on sex per se may be describing needs and wants that are primarily for adventure rather than for sexual variety.

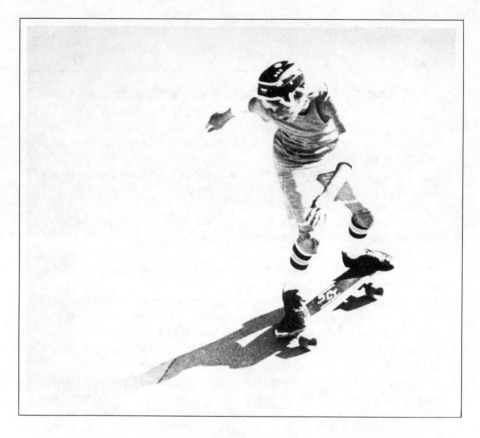

The following exercise will help you to recognize the fantasy stories you create for yourself.

Exercise 5 — Watching Fantasies

1. Give vent to your usual daydreams and fantasies, bringing the "witness state" into play. Remember that "the witness" is an impartial observer, never a judge or censor.

2. Ask yourself, "What does this daydream tell me about what I want or what is missing in my life?"

3. Write the above question down and answer it or share the answer aloud with a friend.

4. Ask yourself what other hidden wants and needs your fantasies reveal. Write these down and/or share them with someone.

Your physical body mirrors that which you think and feel

I am going to suggest a hypothesis: What you think affects what you feel and what you feel affects what you think, and all of this is reflected in your physical body, both inside and outside.

The following exercise will clarify the relationship between what you feel and what you perceive or think.

Exercise 6 — The Eyes of the Beholder

1. Begin by observing whatever it is you are feeling. This can be an emotional feeling or a feeling associated with your physical body.
2. Ask yourself the question: How does this feeling affect my perception and thereby my thinking process?
3. Write your observations down and check out their accuracy with those around you. Keep in mind that you are not judging your process, just observing it. The more impartial good humor you can bring into this experience, the more enlightening it will be for you!

Awareness of that which you feel

Now that you're beginning to observe the patterning of your selective thoughts with a focus on how they affect you in a feeling way, I want to suggest that you enter into the system as an observer from a different point — that is, begin to observe how that which you *feel* affects that which you *think* or perceive. Actually what is really going on is a whole chain of relationships between thoughts and feelings that are not isolated events and therefore have no beginnings or endings. Depending on where you tap into the cycle of events you observe feeling following thought or thought following feeling.

Attitudes provide an example of mental constructs that can influence and sometimes determine emotional states and physical processes. A powerful example would be the attitude people have about the relative friendliness or unfriendliness of the universe. *If the universe is out to get you, the life you lead will be very different from one lived with an expectation of benevolence.* The difference between trust and fear, "thou" and "it" relationships, a mistake that punishes or one that teaches, constructive or destructive criticism, all can be determined by an attitude that views the world as either hostile, indifferent or benevolent.

For example, I note that when I am feeling physically well and emotionally light, it does not trouble me in the least to pass my kids' messy rooms. I see the mess as mess but thoughts along the lines of "after all, the rooms belong to them" come to me and the good mood is sustained. On the other hand, when I am feeling less well physically or emotionally, exactly the same scene elicits anger. For a second or two my thoughts are full of scenes of recrimination and punishment. It's clear to me that in such a situation a qualitative feeling has affected my mental response to a given situation.

Another way of saying this is to point out the inconsistency with which we respond to similar situations. Later in this book, in the Postlude on disease, the correlation between distrust and disease will be more fully explored.

The following exercise will help you to begin perceiving the mirror-like relationship between your body and your thoughts and feelings.

Exercise 7 — My Face — The Mirror of My Inner World

1. Take a good look at your face in the mirror right now. Exactly what do you see? Take a long, careful and detached look. Study with a draftsman's eye the brow, the area around the eyes, the expression in the eyes themselves. How does the left side differ from the right? What about the mouth, the pucker and lines surrounding the mouth? Does it turn up or down, and how does one side differ from the other?

2. Ask yourself the following questions, writing down the answers:
   a. What does this face that is your face suggest or express?
   b. What is its mood?
   c. If you met this face in a crowd, how would you react to it?
   d. Is this a face — an expression — that you would move toward, that you would feel safe with, or is it a face suggestive of fear, pain or distrust?
   e. Is it rested or tired? Tense or relaxed?

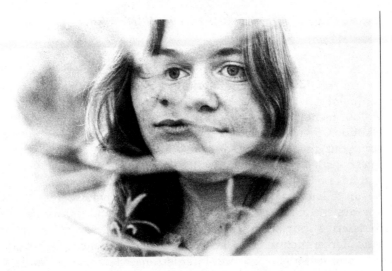

3. Ask yourself and write down the answers to the following questions: Are there places within my body that are directly connected with parts of my face?

    a. Do my eyes or mouth connect to what I experience in my stomach or chest at this minute?

    b. What connection can I make between what I see and what I experience myself thinking and/or feeling?

4. Strip and once more observe with detachment this body that is yours. Again slowly, exactingly and with an attitude of curiosity, not judgment—as if you were an artist with a drawing pen at hand—observe what you see: the bone structure, the musculature, the placement of the head on the neck . . . the positioning of the shoulders, hips, knees, ankles and feet.

5. Ask yourself:

    a. What differences exist between the right and left sides of the body?

    b. What story does this body tell, what experiences and attitudes does this form express?

    c. How does what I see on the surface reflect attitudes and emotions from within?

    d. Is it possible to conceive of the inner structures of this form— tissue, muscle, organs, etc.—as also being expressive of thoughts and emotions?

If you get tired of looking at yourself in the mirror, you might begin to look carefully at others in the same way, verifying whenever possible your assumptions about what feelings, thoughts or attitudes underlie the physical form.

You're on your way!

Stop! Freeze! is the way I put it when I was a kid. Now hold onto the awareness of the moment. Begin playing with it. Observe with discernment what is going on with you internally and externally. Take a look at your mental pictures and processes. Now switch to observing your emotions. Switch again to a focus of yourself in terms of energy. Now scan your physical body for its sensations. To the extent that the above questions have engaged you—if only for an instant—you are *on your way*. You have begun to experience the transformational process. You have begun to know the complex wholeness that is your being. You are not one-dimensional; you are multi-dimensional, and the words that you use to describe yourself in a given moment can only describe one part of a much larger picture. This larger picture I have called the holistic perspective, and it is a personal and interpersonal view that is limitless in its capacity to absorb and expand.

From now one, we will touch on ways and means of opening and extending the incredibly rich and complex being that you represent. If your awareness has been stretched—even a bit—there is no turning back. You're on your way!

Notes to Chapter II

[1] This is an experience that I often use to begin my classes on holistic health.

[2] The witness state is a concept found in the religious philosophies of both East and West. I was first introduced to the idea in undergraduate philosophy studies at U.C.L.A.; later Brugh Joy, a friend and teacher, brought its importance home to me. See *Joy's Way* in the Bibliography. (Each time I refer to a book, I will mention the author and title; see the Bibliography for the publication information on the book and for other books on related subjects.)

[3] Experience teaching this material has shown me that people are far less observant than they realize, and actually remember far less than they believe they do.

[4] See Albert Einstein, *The Meaning of Relativity*, and B. Toben and J. Sarfatti, *Space-Time and Beyond*. The latter is a good general introduction to the new physics for the unscientific.

[5] Two inspiring books on this subject are E. Herrigel, *Zen in the Art of Archery*, and R. Pirsig, *Zen and the Art of Motorcycle Maintenance*. Each in different ways describes this process in depth from an inner perspective.

[6] This information was taken from a class I took with Dr. Jean Houston. See R. Masters and J. Houston, *Mind Games*.

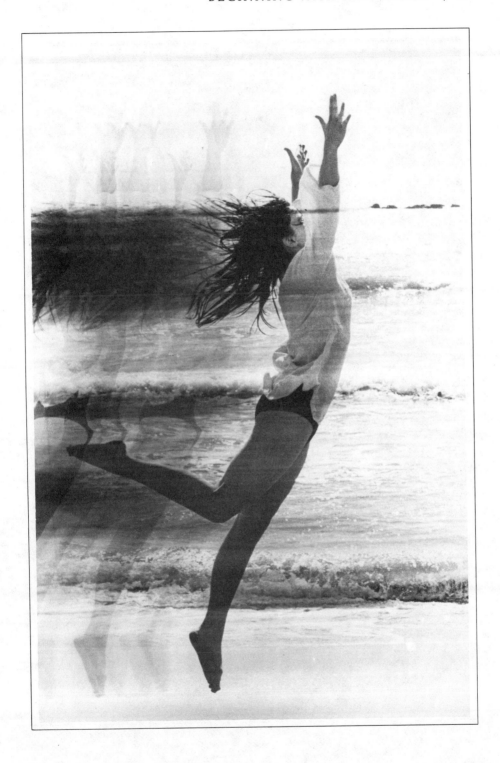

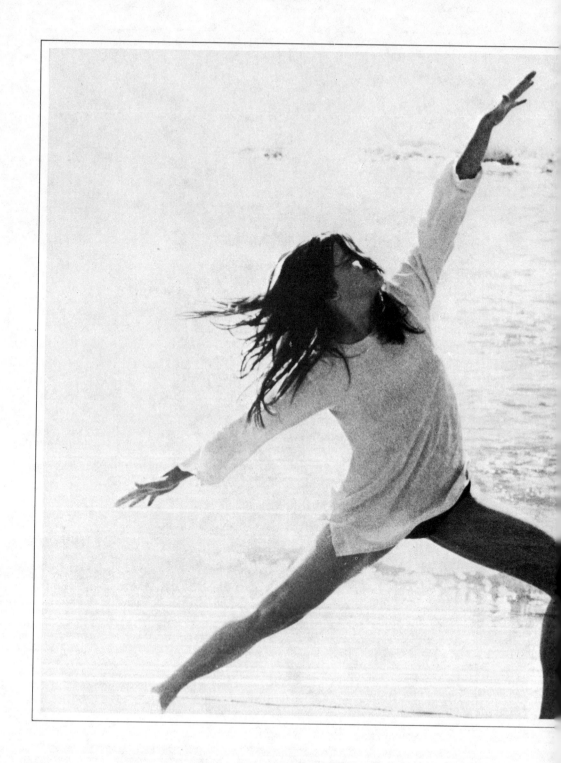

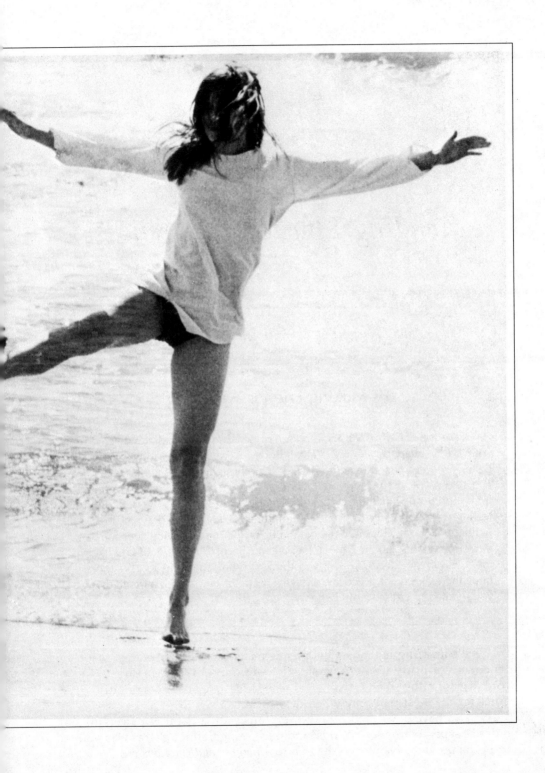

3

Extending Physical Awareness

The following writing exercise will teach you about your body.

Exercise 8—Making Friends with Your Body

Take a piece of paper and a pencil or pen and begin a dialogue with your body.[1] Start by writing, "Dear Body—I want to get to know you better." Write your statement, then let your thoughts go for a moment or two while you give conscious attention to your body. Check yourself from the toes up, including your skin, muscles and viscera. Now let the feeling you experience translate into pictures or words and draw these or write them down. Continue the dialogue, asking the following questions: How do you feel, body? Do you feel taken care of? What would you like me to do or not do for you? If you think of other questions to ask, continue the dialogue as if you were having a conversation with a friend that you wanted to get to know better.

What's amazing is that so few people really regard their bodies as a true friend, and for many it's nothing short of a nuisance. What we do is try to avoid disease rather than learn to feel really well. We take note of our bodies for the most part only when they distress us.

We also have developed into the very misleading habit of perceiving our bodies as separate from our minds[2] and our feelings, although—as was pointed out in the previous chapter—they're not! *Thoughts and emotions etch*

50

themselves into cellular structure and express our life experiences. Individuals trained carefully to observe others can describe what these people have thought about and felt simply by looking at the body's structure. The expressions on people's faces, the way they move and hold themselves suggest very definite attitudes and life experiences.

If thoughts and feelings influence our physical structure, so it is also true that relaxing, extending and improving this form can sharpen our thinking and lift us emotionally.[4] There is a direct relationship, for example, between random movement and brain cell growth.[4] *All kinds of movement in general and random movement in particular sharpen memory and actually make us smarter.* Some creative aging centers aware of this fact have done remarkable work restoring memory and even appearing to reverse senility through programs that have taught the aged to begin moving again in a variety of different ways. Moreover, increased circulatory stimulation — blood moving more rapidly through our bodies — results in a heightened sense of energy and generates an emotional sensation of well-being intense enough to be called "joy." *As far as I am concerned, the best and most reliable "upper" in the world is movement sufficiently difficult or involving to capture and hold attention for ten or twenty minutes.*[5] Aside from being good for you, exercise can be fun. There are countless ways to move that will stretch and strengthen us physically. Some, like aerobics, calisthenics and most games, are vigorous and stimulate the heart and lungs along with the skeletal muscles. Others are performed in a state of relative calm. These include yoga, T'ai Chi, isometrics and the work of Moshe Feldenkrais, to mention a few. All build strength, endurance and flexibility — some more so, depending on the individual, than others. Any kind of exercise is preferable to no exercise, and there is some movement form for everybody. Even the brittle bones of a ninety-year-old can manage the Feldenkrais stretches. The point is to begin now and to begin by acknowledging and loving the body that you have. Conceive of it as a good friend that can provide you with additional energy, vitality and pleasure.

Learning to move

If you're a person who has always enjoyed movement and exercise or enjoyed it at one time, then beginning a physical exercise program is not so difficult. You have all those wonderful memories about how terrific you used to feel. On the other hand, if you have few positive memories or possibly some negative ones, then you may be rationally convinced that movement is a good thing, but you're not very likely to get behind it with the kind of energy it takes to seriously structure a new way of being. If this is the case, my suggestion is to begin with an activity that is already pleasant and familiar to you and bridge it with physical movement. For example, if you love music, dance to it, do yoga, aerobics or calisthenics to whatever kind of music excites and delights you. *Use that which you love to prime yourself for doing that which you don't particularly love—at first!* As your strength increases, the process itself will become its own reward. To begin with, however, you might do well to focus primarily on the music and then on the delicious feelings that follow the experience. In time the process itself will be sufficiently motivating. In this way an old pattern that suggests "my body does not enjoy movement" is replaced by a new pattern or habit that suggests "my body does enjoy it."

The following exercise will acquaint you with this process.

Exercise 9 — Moving to Music

1. Carefully select a piece of music that fills you with the desire to move—to swing and sway or tap your toe, etc.
2. Give yourself time to really focus—don't rush yourself.
3. If you're self-conscious about moving, put a lock on your door.
4. Let the music carry you into the movement form you've chosen. Dance, stretch, twist, lift and bend to the sound and rhythm. Let it energize and inspire you. Nowadays you can even jog to music with earphones!

Music is only one way of bridging an old form with a new one. Perhaps you like to engage in certain daydreams or fantasies—use these to get you going. For centuries people have expressed their love of life, of one another and of God through moving and dancing forms. I think of the Sufi dancing, of Hasidic Jews in a circle, arms around one another in ecstatic movement, and of the Black culture in general when I think of moving forms deeply connected to inner life.

The next exercise is an example of how an inner process is evoked in conjunction with physical movement.

Exercise 10 — Exercise As Spiritual Practice

1. Select a type of exercise that has some appeal for you and, preferably, can be done out-of-doors. Jogging, swimming, tennis, handball, brisk walking, T'ai Chi, yoga, etc., lend themselves to a pairing of the

physical with the spiritual. (In the East the pairing of the physical with the spiritual is accepted as routine.)

2. Now as you begin your run, walk or game, pretend that your skin, the encapsulating sack that separates you from all else, has dissolved. The boundary between you and the world around you no longer

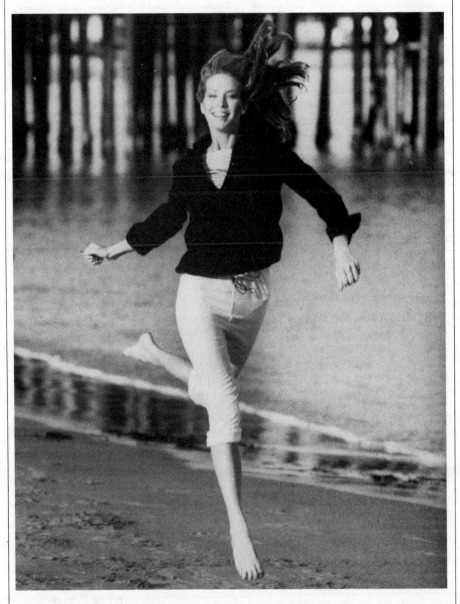

exists. You are at one with the sun, the ball, the trees, the sky. You can't tell where they stop and you begin.

3. Let yourself go and experience the exhilaration that comes with the dissolving of boundaries while you move.

Getting beyond inertia

In addition to bridging the old with the new, there is another technique that can be very helpful in exciting slow starters, and this is to image what it is you want to do before you actually do it.[6] If you want to jump out of bed and start dancing or running, then before you fall asleep, visualize yourself dancing or running joyfully. See yourself feeling pleasure in the experience. Once your brain has begun the moving process electrochemically—which is what happens when you image intensely—then the rest of your body will be able to follow through with much greater ease. The seeding has taken place—the possibility is experienced and you're well on your way even though you haven't as yet begun to physically move.

The following exercise will help you start to move.

Exercise 11—Beginning Exercise for People Who Hate Exercising

1. Before you go to sleep at night, and/or when you awaken in the morning, visualize yourself jumping out of bed and beginning to start the appropriate movements.

2. Involve as many of your senses in this process as you can—touch, taste, smell and hear the experience! Let the imaging be really joyous.

3. Now immediately begin doing what you just visualized, if this is the time you have set aside for "the real thing."

4. Sometimes it's helpful to do the imaging several times during the day as reinforcement for the event.

There are, of course, many ways in which to move. Besides such familiar activities as walking, running and participating in sports, there are the following: (1) *Aerobics*—a form of exercise that stimulates visceral muscles with emphasis on the heart and lungs. One has the choice of carefully paced programs in running, walking, bicycle riding or swimming. This program takes into consideration age, sex and strength, insuring a graduated building of strength and endurance. (2) *Calisthenics*—another physical activity that works very well for many people. Moreover, since there are many group exercise programs available at gyms, YWCAs or YMCAs, community organizations, universities and high schools, etc., this type of movement can be shared with others. People who can't bear to move alone may have a very different experience moving as part of a group. The group energy seems to carry them beyond their individual aversion to physical activity.

Stretch first

You must be careful in any strenuous activity to begin by stretching and limbering up. The need to stretch in order to avoid injury to the muscles, tendons and bones is always present when movement is likely to be strenuous. (See R. Hittleman, *Introduction to Yoga*.) Stretching in order to avoid injury is also advisable before participating in sports activities—tennis, skiing, basketball, etc. "Warming up" properly is important, for we spend so much of our lives physically inactive that it can be a shock to the body to suddenly begin intense movement.

The following exercise will help insure against injuring yourself through strenuous movement.

Exercise 12 — Stretching

1. Very slowly move your head around in a circular fashion, first to the left and then to the right.
2. Slowly stretch each arm up as high as you can, to the side as far as you can and down as far as you can, bending at the waist.
3. Make circles to the left and then the right with your hips.
4. Put your hands on your knees and circle them a few times in one direction and then the other.
5. Lie on your back and circle your ankles in one direction and then the other.
6. While continuing to lie on your back, point your toe and stretch each leg. Now point with your heel and do the same thing.

In addition to the movement classes that can be taken at gyms, there are some newer group forms that aim at gently opening, renewing and extending physical structure. These include the Feldenkrais method and the Alexander technique. Classes like this are especially suitable for the aged and handicapped because they are very gentle, and yet they can be remarkably effective. A form of movement that often appeals to people who are generally resistant to exercise is free-style dancing to music. The "beat" can get you going. It is something you can do rain or shine at any time of day. Moreover, ten to twenty minutes of free-form movement can be very challenging physically as well as a delightful experience. The key for slow starters is to select music to dance to that is so energizing you just can't sit still![5]

Another thing to keep in mind is that no matter what movement form you explore and develop, *any activity repeated again and again in the same way begins to lose its original value.* As soon as a form has become a routine, it's time to vary it or alternate it with others. In this way, the wonderful feeling of physical strength and vigor is maximized and ongoing.

Whatever form moving takes for you, a key factor is awareness. To move and exercise without awareness of what you are doing can actually be harmful. Listen to your body—let it speak to you. Let it tell you how long and far to push it. Care for it—LOVE it! In that way you will not only avoid injuring yourself, but you will be extending your consciousness and expanding your brain as well.

There is more to eating than swallowing

Food dramatically affects your well-being whether you know it or not. It affects the way you feel physically, the way you respond emotionally and the way you perceive mentally. It lifts your energy resource, or sends you plummeting into sleep and unconsciousness. Most people are conscious about food only when it has made them noticeably ill. The question we need to be asking is not, does it make us sick, but rather, *how* well does it make us? *How much better do we feel after we've eaten?* How much more energy, enthusiasm and passion for life do we experience after a meal or a snack? The key when it comes to selecting foods on this basis is again awareness. How do you feel after you swallow the food? How do you feel in five minutes, in an hour, after several hours, and how do you feel generally?

The following exercise will help you to track well-being in relationship to what you eat.

Exercise 13 — The Relationship between Food and Feeling

1. Eat in your usual way. Select the foods and the times for eating that you normally do, adding to this process awareness of what you are doing.

2. Make a chart or a log of *all* that you eat, including in-between nibbles and snacks. Don't kid yourself — you won't remember it all unless you write "it all" down!

3. Pay attention to your feelings, physical and emotional — five minutes after you have eaten; one hour after you have eaten; two or three hours after you have eaten.

Notice if there has been a shift or change as the result of eating. Do you feel better or worse than before you ate? Do you feel energized or tired? How well has eating made you feel?

4. Keep this process up for at least three days a week.

Keeping the above chart or log will heighten your awareness tenfold even if you think you know what the answers are without keeping a log. The consciousness that results from in-the-moment experience is much more effective and has more impact than any other.

Making yourself knowledgeable about the great variety of nutritional theories and practices is a part of that responsibility which again, in the end, means a careful attunement to the way foods and food groups affect individual well-being. *Fortunately, your own body can truly be counted on to tell you what is needed.* The more attuned you are to your body and the better you care for it, the more this is the case.

There is an often repeated experiment done on ten-month-old babies where they are given an opportunity to choose freely from all the food groups. They eat whatever they want in the amounts they want, and while they may binge on one food or another for a short time, within a few days it becomes apparent that over and over again, relying entirely on instinctual hungers, nutritious and balanced choices have been made. Babies, of course, really do consult their stomachs before beginning to eat or asking for more.

When the question repeatedly asked is, "How well do I feel after a meal or snack?" the process of gaining awareness of nutritional needs is underway. An increase in energy and an expanded feeling of well-being become nutritional barometers. The purpose of eating shifts from the intention to feel full of food to the intention to feel full of energy and

The following exercise will sensitize you to the effect food combinations and quantities have on your well-being.

Exercise 14 — Mixing and Matching Foods

1. Begin to experiment with your food:
   a. Try eating less food more often, or less, period.
   b. If you're a meat-eater, spend two or three days excluding meat from your diet.
   c. Perhaps you will want to exclude red meat, but include chicken and/or fish.
   d. Delete certain foods from your diet: salt, sugar, coffee and bread, for example, and see how this affects your well-being.
   e. Play with food combinations. Try eating solely starch meals or protein meals, or fruit meals or vegetable meals.

2. Keep a chart or log of all that you observe in yourself as you experiment with your eating practices. The question you're researching is "which eating patterns add to the quality of life, and which don't?"

3. Continue this assessment on the basis of kinds, combinations and amounts of food you eat for two or three weeks.

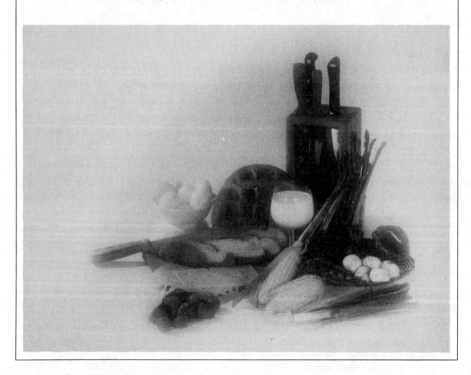

well-being. A nutritional "glutton" wants to feel *full* of energy as much as possible, and selects foods and food combinations that support this intention. When this is what is wanted, increased awareness is facilitated by slowing down at mealtimes.

As awareness grows, it becomes apparent that much food consumption has nothing to do with physical hunger and everything to do with calming, soothing and pacifying. In other words, the well-being that many seek through eating is connected to something other than the need to fill

The following exercise will help you to slow down at mealtimes and increase awareness of what you are doing.

Exercise 15 — Eating in Slow Motion

1. Imagine yourself, as you normally eat, projected on a movie screen.
2. Rewind the film and turn the projector to "slow motion." Visualize, sense and feel yourself moving very slowly this time on the screen as you select and eat. Taste in slow motion!
3. Repeat this visualization when you awaken each morning and once or twice during the day.

This exercise will serve as a reminder and reinforce the intention to change focus from ingesting to awareness.

our hungry stomachs. Food is a stand-in for, among other things, love and sex in this culture. Filling, saturating oneself with foods, stills for a short time other kinds of hunger. Lonely people often eat a lot. The irony is that consciousness, clarity of mind and perception are dulled in the process of eating, and so the real hungers are overlooked. It is painful to be hungry and to know it . . . painful in the sense that one knows something is wanted that is not at hand, painful in the sense that going after what one wants may be difficult and risky. Pain in this sense is difficult, but instructive. It is a message that has been received — you are wanting something, you are needing something, and the discomfort is a reminder to attend to that which is wanted and needed.

For example, what an individual may crave after dinner may be some activity that's challenging or exciting, or it may be a release from the pressure of the day's stress. The craving, however, takes the form in consciousness of a "little something to nibble on." This "something that's needed" may be physical, psychological, mental or spiritual. When people dull awareness with food, they overlook and thereby discount their own needs. *Once food is connected to physical well-being rather than emotional well-being, the process of food selection becomes one of careful listening to your own body.* For example, you may find that when you eat proteins you feel heavy and sluggish for hours. Protein, then, or a lot of protein, becomes something for you, personally, to more or less avoid. On the other hand, even though you may have made a mental decision to be vegetarian, you will reverse that decision if upon really listening to your body you find yourself feeling hungry or low energy much of the time. The point is that the nutritious selection of food is individual and determined by many factors, including genetic inheritance, lifestyle, the amount and kind of work we do, the environment, etc. This same principle applies when it comes to deciding whether or not to take vitamins and supplements. Energy and a heightened sense of well-being is what we are after. The way you feel when you take vitamins and supplements will tell you whether or not your particular body needs them. Of course, this places the responsibility for choosing what to eat, how much to eat, and in what combinations *squarely upon you.*

The following exercise also increases awareness of eating.

Exercise 16 — Pausing to Enjoy Your Food

1. Begin by taking a deep breath.
2. Check your body to insure that it's relaxed. (Refer to exercises described in the section on stress beginning a few pages further on in this book.)
3. Ask yourself the question, "What is it that I am really hungry for? Is it food? What kind of food? How hungry am I?"
4. Continue to ask these questions throughout the meal.

When you eat selectively, you eat only that which you truly want, and in the amount you want it. Be prepared to surprise yourself in terms of what you will discover.[6]

Snacking on breath, or breath as food

One of the most amazing and delightful discoveries I've made in relationship to hunger has to do not with food as we normally think of it, but rather with breath. Breathing deeply pacifies hunger . . . not in every situation, of course, or totally, but dependably, and to a degree that never ceases to surprise me. Oxygen, like food, fuels the body, and fresh, clean air deeply breathed serves a food-like function in that it assuages hunger while providing increased energy and a sense of well-being. Oxygen is probably a fuel source that all of us who lead urban lives are deficient in.

I believe that the gnawing hunger many city dwellers experience expresses the body's deep need for this particular kind of fuel. Have you ever noticed, for example, that exercise leaves you less, rather than more, hungry?

The following exercise will make you aware of the filling quality of breath.

Exercise 17 — Taking a Bite of Breath

1. Whenever you feel hungry, and before every meal, take ten slow, deep breaths. (Refer to Exercise 21 if you wish.)
2. Reflect on what it is you really want.

I wish that I could take credit for this marvelous discovery, but I understand that Indian holy men and many others, too, no doubt, have known about the nutritional aspect of breath for centuries. In this regard, the most nutritious breath is that which fills you with fresh, clean air, and my preference is to feast in this manner surrounded by sunshine, so that the smell of fresh air and the warmth of the sun have become reminders to fill up deeply with oxygen. Of course, as you breathe deeply you also relax stress and tension — a common initiator of false hunger.

Stress, or what do do after the horse is already out of the barn

Stress is a word that's hard to escape from hearing these days. It is often used as the catchall — the bad guy for whatever is wrong with us physically or emotionally, the reason the body breaks down and is unable to defend itself against disease, the provocation for neurosis, and often psychosis. If we weren't stressed so much of the time we would probably feel terrific much more often, and live well beyond our normal life expectencies! Therefore, in extending our bodies we have to extend our consciousness of stress.[7]

Basically, I define stress as a physiological response to a psychological event, and that event is *change*. In cultures where life has a prescribed routine, and nothing much interferes with that routine year in and year

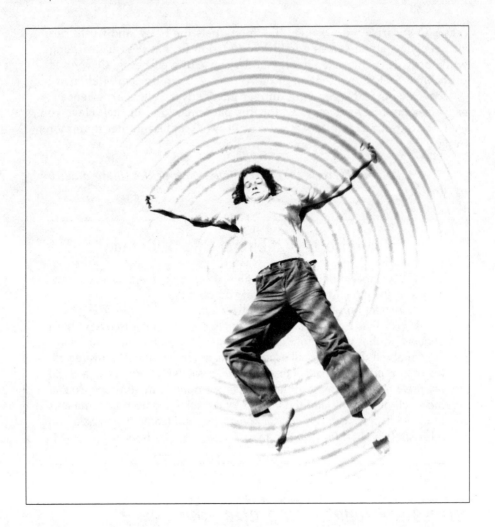

out for generations, people do not have that experience of life called stress. In cultures like ours, however, change is inevitable. The environment, for example, we all know to be fluctuating rapidly. The air we breathe and the nutrients in the food we eat are qualitatively different from that of food eaten and air breathed thirty-five years ago. In addition to external change, many of us lead lives of internal discontinuity. Jobs begin and end, friendships and relationships come and go, whole lifestyles shift when people divorce, retire or change jobs. In the flick of an eye the continuity of being is shattered for a time. Change in this fast-moving culture is inevitable, and much of it is evidently beyond our control.

Added to this are the changes we ourselves choose in order to improve the quality of life. So much more is available to us, so much more possible than a generation or two ago. This book is a part of that emerging trend of thought that says you can choose and change your way of being, and I know this to be true. I also know that moving toward increased "well-being" represents a fundamental change for many people, a change that is stressful emotionally and physiologically, and has therefore to be acknowledged and accounted for.[8]

The beginning point is the recognition and acknowledgement of the difficulty involved in shifting behavior patterns, even those that move us in the direction of increased pleasure and satisfaction. We are moving from that which is known to that which is unknown, and *few people possess the kind of self-trust that makes the unknown truly safe.* The great dilemma for people who seek a fuller experience of life is the fear of change experienced both physically and emotionally as stress.

Resolution lies in honoring both sides: the need to explore, evolve and alter established patterns, and the concurrent need for continuity. The question for contemporary explorers is, *"How do I build sufficient continuity into my life to enable me to explore and evolve without self-destructing?"* Unfortunately, the patterns that support us in this way are often long-standing, and inappropriate. And sometimes they're in direct opposition to our chosen evolutionary path. Many people give their lives continuity with negative forms—eating when they're not hungry, addiction to TV or anything else and even emotional states like anger, depression or irritability. *Many old habits continue to serve us as familiar agents of continuity until we consciously create others that are more constructive. It is important, therefore, consciously to select a group of patterns and behaviors that are constructive, satisfying and ongoing.* Such patterns deeply "de-stress us," giving us periods in our fluctuating, fast-moving lives of at-oneness with ourselves, other people and the universe. A number of different practices can meet this need. Exercise is one of these. (See the suggestions earlier in this chapter.) Another is meditation.

Meditation

In meditation, the thoughts, cares and concerns of the moment are surrendered, while the body is focused on and subsequently de-stressed. A great variety of meditative forms have been introduced in the last few years.[9] A meditative form, like a food, varies in its effectiveness from person to person, and even with the same person when times and circumstances change. There are a number of very simple meditative forms that anyone can use immediately. Any of the following can help you to quiet yourself, relax, de-stress and turn your attention from that which is outside of you to that which is within you. The inner focus characteristic of all meditations balances and refreshes. It is also capable of leading eventually to profound states of awareness and inspiration.

A rule of thumb for beginners in meditation has to do with creating a special time and space for yourself in order to de-stress. That is, create an attractive place for yourself in your home or office and insure its sacredness or specialness by taking responsibility for not being interrupted. This means no telephones to answer or people running in to distract you. Meditations don't have to be long. Ten minutes can work wonders, so don't be afraid to put a lock on the door or a "Please Do Not Disturb" sign. I was able to take ten minutes for myself in this way, even when my children were very young.

The following exercise will introduce you to simple meditations.

Exercise 18 — Beginning Steps to Meditation

1. Select a special time and place for your meditation. Plan to give yourself ten to twenty minutes of uninterrupted time. Experienced meditators often prefer a time frame of from forty-five minutes to one hour. There is, however, no "right" amount of time or frequency for meditation. Begin with what you're comfortable with and proceed from there.

2. Sit or lie with your back straight. You can sit in a chair or on the floor. For those not used to sitting quietly erect for some time, a pillow or two can make you more comfortable. If you choose to lie down, you take the chance of falling asleep. Sleep is fine, but it is *not* meditation!

3. Focus your attention on your body. Do you detect tightness or discomfort anywhere? If you do, try to relax and release these areas by tensing them first and then letting go. Breathing into the areas of tension —using your imagination to send the streams of your breath through them—is also effective.

4. Select one of the following meditative styles and make the choice to follow it for a time:

    a. Following Your Breath[11]

        1. Sit quietly and relax, with your spine erect, for ten to twenty minutes, just following your breath. Give your full attention to the inhalation-exhalation process—nothing more. Allow thoughts that come into your head to pass through, returning each time this happens to the focus on your breath.

        2. If your concentration lags don't allow this to upset you, simply refocus and continue.

    b. Repeating a Sound[12]

1. Sit quietly relaxed for from ten to twenty minutes, giving undivided attention to a word, a sound or a group of sounds that you repeat over and over again silently to yourself, or aloud if you prefer. The vowel sounds, a, e, i, o, u, or the "do, re, mi" of the scale are useful examples of words or sounds that can be used in this way. Traditional meditative sounds such as "Om-m-m" or "ah-h-h" can also be selected, or you may want to make yours up.

2. If distracting thoughts interrupt your concentration, do not get upset, just refocus and continue.

c. Contemplating a Crystal, Flower, etc.

1. Select an object of interest and beauty that attracts your attention.

2. Sit quietly, spine erect, for from ten to twenty minutes, gazing at the object. Give it your complete, undivided attention.

3. If distracting thoughts pass through your mind, accept them and let them go.

d. Meditating to Music

1. Select a piece of music that inspires you, lifts you and holds your attention. Classical music is particularly good for meditative pusposes. (Most music stores carry tapes and records of music especially created for meditations.)

2. Lie on the floor, palms down, and listen to the music with the volume turned up to a comfortable level.

3. Let yourself melt into the sound. Become the sound. Let it lift and carry and engage you completely.

4. If you have an emotional response to the music, allow it.

5. If thoughts interfere with your concentration, don't get upset, just refocus and continue.

Calming the mind

I've been describing some of the things that one can do in order to relax, de-stress and come around to oneself. The chief thing that you don't do is engage in characteristic thought patterns. In other words, you don't think your usual thoughts in the usual way. You surrender them for a brief time—knowing full well that they'll be waiting for you. Your intention is to quiet thoughts, to relax them and to let them go. Personally, I've always found this extremely difficult to do. Combining strenuous exercise with meditation was helpful to me in this regard. Any form of vigorous movement will probably allow you to sit quietly without thinking for a more extended period of time than you're used to.

The following exercises will help you to quiet your chattering mind.

Exercise 19 — Moving/Sitting Meditation[14]

1. Spend ten to twenty minutes dancing, shaking, hopping, running, swimming, etc., *actively.*

2. Now sit quietly, spine erect, for from ten to twenty minutes.

3. Concentrate on what your body feels like. Relax and focus on your physical sensations.

You can also quiet your mind through visualization. Visualizations can take many forms. Some people go in their imaginations to the mountains or seashore, to a cave deep in the earth or to outer space. The more you engage your senses in this imaging process, the more likely you will be to successfully disengage your thoughts and relax. Therefore, sense — feel, smell, see, hear, touch, taste — the imaginary scene.

Exercise 20 — Calming Your Overactive Mind

1. Sit erect and relaxed, imagining your mind chatter personified as a distraught baby or a yelping puppy.

2. Tenderly engage as many of your senses as you can to calm and soothe it. Rock and sing to it, but don't let your mind fall asleep, because then you will!

3. Let your mind be both peaceful and alert.

You need not, by the way, be a visualizer in order to image. Simply activate those senses that are available to you. For example, you can hear, taste or smell a scene without ever seeing it.

Deep full breathing

One of the simplest and yet most effective de-stressing practices is to breathe smoothly, deeply and fully. By this, I mean an inhalation sufficient to fill both the stomach and chest — simultaneously or alternately stomach/chest or chest/stomach.

The following exercise will teach you to send oxygen to both your chest and belly.

Exercise 21—Chest/Belly Breathing

1. Lie down in front of a mirror with an unobstructed view of your chest and stomach.

2. Put one hand on your stomach and the other on your chest so that you can both see and feel your breathing.

3. Breathe in deeply, filling *both* your belly and chest. Either can be filled with oxygen first—chest/belly or belly/chest, or they can be filled simultaneously.

4. Try to take ten full, smooth breaths this way every day for a week or two, and you'll soon catch the rhythm.

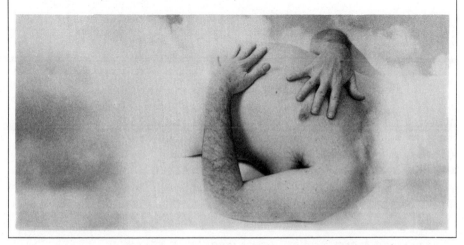

If you're like most people, you will have found filling both chest and stomach with oxygen difficult if not downright impossible to do. That's OK, keep trying. It's well worth the effort because what you'll find, once you're able to deeply and smoothly fill your chest and belly, is that it's impossible to be physically tense while doing this. Talk about cheap and effective tranquilizers! In a way, full breathing is for most people also a meditation in that we are so unused to doing it that the practice fully engages our mind. While our bodies are de-stressed and energized with oxygen, our minds are calmed at the same time. Keep in view that this is a natural breathing pattern. We all as infants tended to breathe this way. Once you're able to take full, smooth breaths lying down on the floor, practice doing the same thing from a sitting or standing position, and in this way you can build into your daily life a series of brief, but very effective breathing exercises that de-stress and energize.

Meditation, deep full breathing and exercise, as described in the preceding sections, are only three possibilities for building life-enhancing habits into daily life. Habits or routine practices that quiet the mind, de-stress, relax and energize are limitless in their possibilities. Any practice or activity that we engage in regularly and has a calming effect will do. We can de-stress alone or with another. We can quiet an anxious mind caught up in concern and countless changes and challenges that confront and often seem to assault us by exercising, meditating, gardening, dancing, cooking, housekeeping, model-car building, etc.

Meditation can take place once a day or several times a day. My own preference is to have several short meditations during the day, but I usually settle for one. The more stress we're under, for positive or negative reasons — and very positive experiences like falling in love or receiving a promotion can be highly stressful — the more we need the kind of continuity meditative forms provide.

Laughter

Laughter is another example — one of the most delightful — of a habit or practice that, again, calms, relaxes and deeply de-stresses.[15] A sense of humor and a ready laugh are probably more healing to body and mind than any medication we know of. When we laugh, our perception shifts. We let go feelings of judgment, blame and self-pity to embrace a more extended knowing of ourselves and others. Deliberately taking the time to amuse and be amused allows us to sustain a great deal of change that would otherwise be overwhelming.

The following exercise will promote laughter in your life.

Exercise 22 — Learning to Laugh

1. Make it a point to spend time with people who make you laugh and do it regularly.

2. Learn to play like a child and be silly. Taking an improvisational theatre class can be helpful. Or make friends with a very young person. Babies and young children haven't forgotten how to laugh and play. Let them be your teachers!

3. Many wonderful books have been written around the subject of humor. Check these out of the library and read them — preferably aloud, sharing with others. One person's laughter evokes another's.

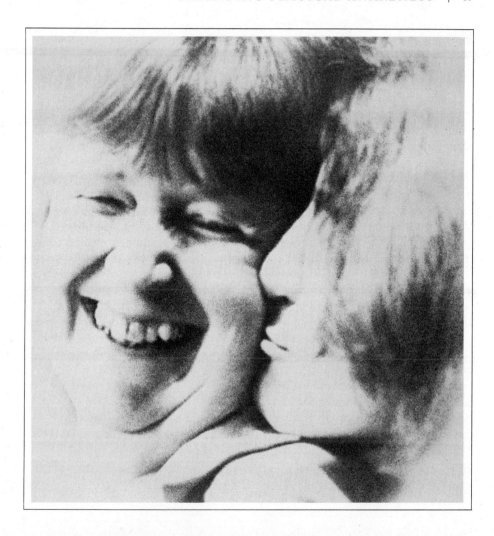

The practice of touching, holding and being held is another habit that can permit us to undergo change in a balanced way. Much stress and tension may be resolved this way. People who are affectionate and aware come to realize that the practice of touching and embracing others has as much to do with calming themselves as it does loving others.

There are many ways to de-stress, to calm, turn inward and relax ourselves. The habits that I have suggested in this section are all life-enhancing. As I said earlier, *many times we build continuity into our lives with habits that may not be life-enhancing, such as depression or compulsiveness.* These patterns can give continuity to living, but often there is a social or personal price to pay that leads to some form of disease. As we become more and more conscious of stress and the patterns that de-stress us, we extend our capacity for change and evolution.

Sexuality—an inexhaustible source of energy

You are about to begin a journey that can only add to your experience of life. The extension of sexual awareness brings with it increased energy, vitality, creativity and enthusiasm for living—all of which can be directed with intention and clarity in countless ways.[18]

Many view sexual energy in terms of a narrow frame of reference that includes genital excitation and little else. Sex from this perspective becomes something that one does rather than something that one is. The focus is on action and activity. Questions of performance, of how often, how to and with whom become those that occupy our attention. Morality—good and bad, right and wrong—enters in and the deeper experience of a sexual life force is obscured in the advice and argument that ensue. It bears repeating to say that *sexuality is a way of being, not merely a way of doing,* and the awareness of this fact brings with it access to an ongoing source of vitality. We are all sexual all of the time, although we do not choose to focus on this aspect of our being all of the time. Just as our heart beats continually whether or not we choose to pay attention to it, so that energy, which derives from the aspect of your humanity called sexuality, generates continuously, and what we do with it—which includes ignoring it—will profoundly affect the way we perceive and experience life. It can be an initiating factor in all kinds of disease (dis-ease), be our disease emotional or physical. Or it can be a source of energy contributing to the quality of life and well-being.

The following exercise is a good one to appraise sexual awareness.

Exercise 23—Tuning in to Sexual Energy

1. Begin by breathing deeply (refer to Experience 21), only this time let the oxygen penetrate your pelvis and fill your genitals.[19]
2. Do this very slowly ten times.
3. Reflect on what is happening to you in your genitals and what you are experiencing generally. Remember to suspend judgment while you observe yourself in the experience.

After this exercise people report feelings that range from pleasure, surprise, an increased sense of energy and quickening to anger, shame and disgust. Some are unable to identify any feeling or sensation at all.

EXTENDING PHYSICAL AWARENESS | 71

The thing to keep in mind is that whatever you are discovering is perfectly all right. Sexual response often varies during the monthly cycle for women. Men too may vary from month to month, so that you may want to spot-check with this exercise over the following month or months.

For those fortunate people who grew up in environments where sexual interest and exploration was regarded as natural and appropriate, one part of life, but not the central focus of life, sexuality is familiar and comfortable. It's neither a big deal nor a little deal. It's there providing for them a wellspring of energy that deepens and enriches life, and fuels everything they do. What if, however, you haven't been so blessed, and when you breathe into your genitals you feel nothing, or something more uncomfortable yet! The thing to keep in mind, no matter what, including age, is that you *are* sexual—awareness of this fact may have dropped below your level of consciousness, but it is there waiting to be brought back into awareness.

Keep in mind too the principle of change in relation to stress as you expand your sexual consciousness. Be gentle and undemanding of yourself as you pursue a path that will extend you sexually.

Using physical exercise to ignite sexuality

There are some very simple physical exercises that ignite sexual awareness and increase genital sensation.

The following exercise will produce greater control and sensitivity in your genitals.

Exercise 24 — Push Pull

1. Scan your body to see if you are holding tension anywhere. If you are, release it. (Refer to de-stressing exercises.)
2. Focus on your genitals, breathing into them.

3. Tense or squeeze your genitals and then relax them.
   a. Squeeze *very* slowly to a count of ten.
   b. Squeeze rapidly in a strobe-like manner up to a count of fifty.
4. Breathe deeply again and pay attention to the feelings in your genitals.
5. Several times during the day try to recall this sensation.

Using visualization to ignite sexuality

Another way of igniting sexual energy and awareness is through visualization. Evocative pictures and sexual fantasy have long been used to evoke sexuality. There are in addition a host of subtler, less overt visualization practices that gently open and expand sexual self-awareness.

The following exercise will give you an example of how this might take place.

Exercise 25 — Visualizing a Bud Opening

1. Check your body to see if it's tense anywhere. If it is, let the tension go.
2. Music is an option in this exercise. If it allows you to relax more deeply, use it.
3. Imagine yourself in a lush field of flowers on a perfect day. Bring all of your senses into play. Feel the warmth of the sun and the coolness of the breeze. See if you can visualize all the color that surrounds you. Sense, taste and touch the scene.
4. Now find a bud among the flowers that's especially beautiful. Let it symbolize your sexuality.
5. Feel the bud in place of your genitals and experience its opening. Feel the sensitive petals part, embracing the warmth of the sun. See its beauty, touch it, smell its perfume.
6. Continue to stay relaxed for a few minutes and enjoy the process.
7. Repeat this visualization at least once a day for at least two weeks upon awakening or just before bed. The longer you continue to practice, the more your sexual awareness will increase.

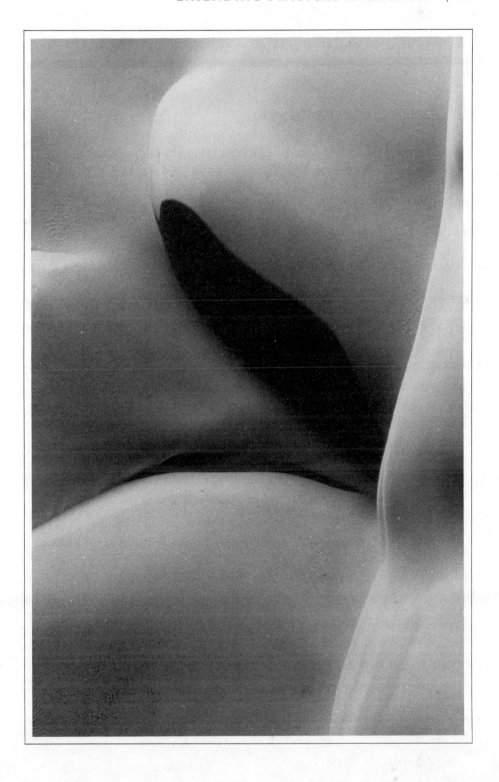

Evoking sexuality through music and dance

The use of music and dance to evoke sexual energy has been around as long as human civilization. Hip-swaying, pulsing rhythms have since time immemorial sparked and awakened slumbering sexuality. If you are having trouble identifying energy that is sexual within you, take a hula or belly-dancing class! Societies that seek to downplay or extinguish sexual awareness permit very little physical movement and discourage those undulating rhythms that do encourage it! One of the reasons why movement is so evocative is that when moving we are forced to breathe fully and deeply. Shallow breathing or breathing that does not move oxygen into the stomach and pelvis diminishes conscious awareness in these parts of our body. When we don't *want to feel* much, what do we do? Hold our breath!

The following exercise uses movement and dance rhythms to spark awareness of sexual feeling.

Exercise 26 — Moving to the Beat

1. Arrange or move the furniture so that you can move freely through the space you have available. If you're the self-conscious type, you might want to lock your door.

2. Select a piece of music that invites you to move and sway your hips.

3. Focus on the rhythm or "beat" rather than the quality of the sound or musical form.

4. Become the rhythm—the instrument being played. Let yourself be at one with it.

5. When the music stops, lie down on your back immediately, palms down and feet stretched out. Focus on your pelvis, and the area that surrounds it.

6. Breathe slowly and deeply and give the feeling in your pelvis your full attention for a few minutes.

7. Allow whatever emotions may come to be expressed. Let yourself laugh, cry—whatever you are moved to do.

The following exercise uses classical music to evoke the generation of earthly energy.

Exercise 27 — Letting the Music Do the Work

1. Get from a library, borrow or buy a copy of Ravel's *Bolero* or Rimsky-Korsakov's *Scheherazade*. (Classical works are given as examples only because I am more familiar with these. An enduring jazz piece would do just as well if you don't care that much for classical music.)

2. Turn up the volume to a comfortable level and lie, palms down, on your back, letting the sound reverberate throughout your body. Become the music. Let it play you.

   a. Release whatever thought patterns are habitually familiar to you. Let them go!
   b. If you should start to feel anxious, breathe deeply and trust the appropriateness of the energies you're experiencing.

3. As the sound dies away, pay attention to all that you are experiencing. Notice that if you have moved deeply into the music the whole of your body has been affected.

All art forms, not only music and dance, are capable of igniting or tapping into sexual energy. A poem, a line, a sculpture, a jazz or symphonic work, as well as forms from nature, have the capacity to awaken in an instant that which may have been slumbering for some time. The possibility of our being ignited in this way is determined by the degree to which we will focus intensely on these art forms, letting go our mental control and thereby allowing the ignition to take place.

Sexuality is a quality of energy that generates from the lower parts of our body, but can be experienced in every cell and pore. This energy is not confined to the pelvis — it only originates there. Its drive is creative, and explorative, and to the extent that procreation is creative and explorative, procreation is an appropriate direction for it. But sexual energy can be, and is, appropriately expressed in many other ways as well. It's the fire that releases an aging musician's arthritic fingers — the drive behind new processes and new projects of all kinds. It is an energy owned by creative, adventuresome people, no matter what their age. Like a car, sexual energy can take us many places, including those we think of as being exclusively mental or spiritual.

I once spent an afternoon with a community of nuns discussing sexuality. This enlightened, intelligent and creative group understood that even though they had made decisions to be celibate, the energy of their sexuality was valuable to them in their creative and spiritual work. They were full of excitement, enthusiasm and playfulness. Rather than deny its existence, they were owning and acknowledging their sexuality—and were thereby in a position to purposefully direct it.[18]

By being sexual, you tap into a resource that can carry you into the bedroom but also, and just as appropriately, into creative expression, and into the world of ideas and spirit.

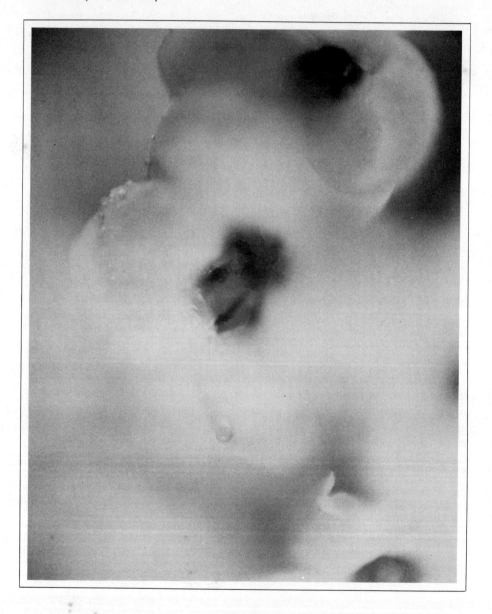

Notes to Chapter III

[1]This is an exercise first introduced to me by my tutor, Dr. Harold Stone.

[2]The research of Dr. Robert Masters and Dr. Jean Houston support this statement. See R. Masters and J. Houston, *Mind Games.*

[3]I have worked with dozens of students and clients, creating individual exercise programs that people were able to stick to. The key is not to insist that everyone do the same thing, or in the same way.

[4]Dr. Jean Houston introduced me to this information. The process is similar to autogenics or self-hypnosis.

[5]For more information on movement, see K. H. Cooper, *The New Aerobics;* W. Barlow, *The Alexander Technique;* Boston, *Our Bodies Ourselves;* R. Hittleman, *Introduction to Yoga;* B. K. S. Iyengar, *Light on Yoga;* M. Feldenkrais, *Awareness Through Movement.*

[6]All of the material in this section on nutrition evolved from the classes I gave on weight control at Everywoman's Village. Experience has led me to believe that general statements about what people should or should not eat are irresponsible. For example, I have known people to so limit salt in the diet as to make themselves ill. What I practice in regard to personal food selection, which is similar to a vegetarian diet, is not what I preach to all I see.

[7]See B. Brown, *New Mind, New Body;* M. Friedman and R. H. Rosenman, *Type A Behavior and Your Heart;* O. C. Simonton and S. S. Simonton, "Belief Systems and Management of the Emotional Aspects of Malignancy," *Journal of Transpersonal Psychology,* 1975, pp. 29–47.

[8]Experience teaching people to integrate process into their lives has taught me this. There is a much greater chance that the learning will be maintained when de-stressing is built into the process of learning.

[9]The material that follows represents a simplification and synthesis of the concepts developed in the books listed under the heading "Meditations" in the Bibliography, plus those I learned working with Dr. Brugh Joy. See W. B. Joy, *Joy's Way.*

[10]I have worked at the Center for the Healing Arts and with private clients now for two years teaching these simplified forms of meditation as an adjunct to psychological counseling.

[11]See E. Herrigel, *Zen.*

[12]See L. Keys, *Toning.*

[13]See R. Dass, *Journey of Awakening: A Meditator's Guidebook.*

[14]See B. Rajneesh, *Meditation: The Art of Ecstasy.*

[15]See N. Cousins, *Anatomy of an Illness as Perceived by the Patient.*

[16]The material in this subsection was explored and developed in classes in sexuality that I taught at Everywoman's Village.

[17]See J. Rosenberg, *Total Orgasm.*

[18]Work with seriously ill people at the Center for the Healing Arts leaves me with the impression that there is definitely a correlation between sexual awareness as I have defined it and breast cancer.

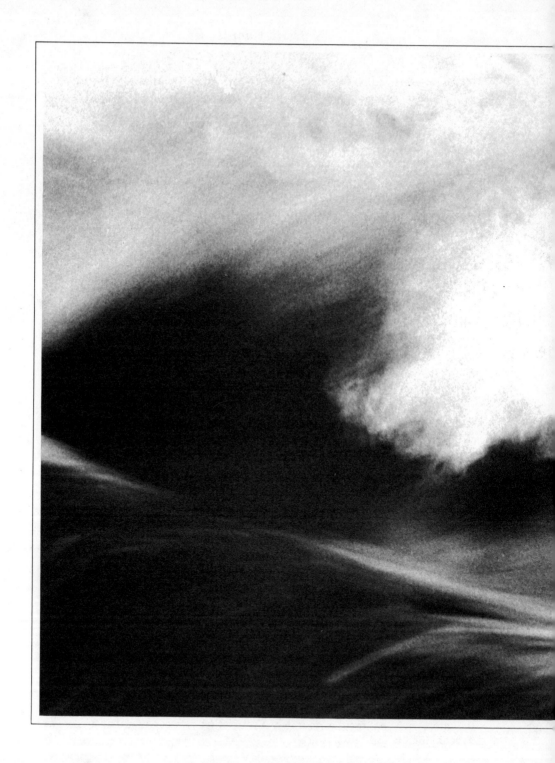

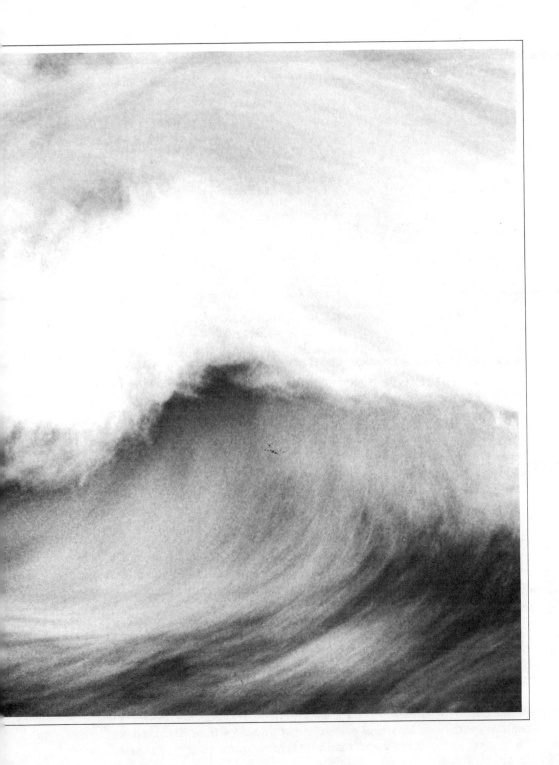

4

Extending Emotional Awareness

Getting to know all about me

An artist friend and I have been engaged in an ongoing dialogue in which she argues that she does not want anyone tampering with her psyche — including herself! What is not conscious and apparent she does not want to know about. Her position is something like the following: Why open up a can of worms? Things that I don't know about might interfere with my life and my work were I to become aware of them. What I don't know doesn't hurt me! Her position expresses the deep fear of the unknown that many people feel, and the belief that those parts of ourselves hidden from awareness are inconsequential in their effect on us. It just does not work that way! Closing our eyes to that which we do not want to see does not make it go away, it just puts us in the position of being more vulnerable standing there in the dark!

Moreover, *if our stated objective is to be whole — all that we are — then settling for less self-understanding is simply not good enough.* Delegating aspects of our personalities to unconsciousness results in a loss of self and thereby a loss of self-choice. Eventually, this leads to some form of dis-ease! Science underscores philosophy here by assuring us that nothing which we experience or feel is ever forgotten or lost by the brain. It's just a question of where the information is stored.

We store information where we can get at it consciously, or we store information where we cannot get at it consciously. In either case, the thoughts, feelings, desires, etc., affect that which we think, feel and do. The more we are able to bring into awareness, the more we understand and have conscious choice in this process.

The exploration of personality is facilitated by being in contact with other people. The "gristfulness" of relationship — intense interaction with others — tends to ignite those aspects of ourselves that lie hidden from consciousness. This is not to say that we can't gain insight on our own, but it is self-deceptive to ignore the limitations of emotional and psychological exploration by oneself.

Emotionally close and intimate contact with others can ignite feelings within us that are frightening or hurtful. For example, we may recall experiences in our past where we were hurt by parents, lovers or children. These emotions are often much easier to ignore when we're alone, particularly if we're occupied with work that's involving. The good reason again for choosing to explore that which may be difficult is that it operates within us, limiting our health and well-being, whether we recognize it or not.

Intimacy — a reflection of myself

There is no way to fully explore emotional awareness apart from intense interaction with other people.[7] We can hone our bodies, stretch our brain-mind systems and explore expanded states of consciousness without involving ourselves with others. However, when we choose to shut down existence in one part of life, we limit all of life to some extent.

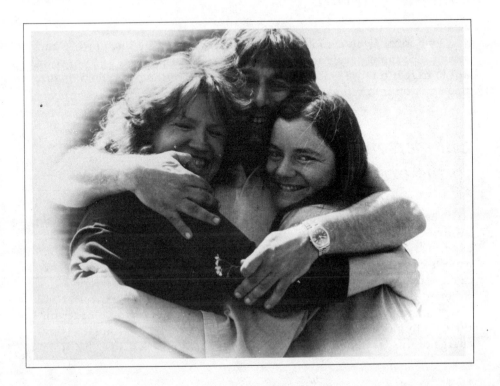

Close and intimate relationships with others ignite and expose our vulnerability. This awareness may not always be pleasant and often we fear that such knowledge will be very unpleasant. *When we don't choose to blame ourselves, knowledge of vulnerability is comfortable.*

Moreover, self-acceptance and understanding brings with it wonderful rewards, including an increase in energy and creative output, the capacity to experience love more fully and an intensification of the joyous and beautiful aspects of life.

A deeply revealing mirror is held up when we become intensely involved with other people, a mirror helping us to experience, often for the first time, those aspects of our personalities most hidden from conscious awareness. That which we may have been able to bury for years is suddenly uncovered. Perhaps, for example, we have thought of ourselves as tough and able to completely forego the love and support of others. A close relationship can punch holes in our toughness, revealing a softness and vulnerability that can appear frightening! Nonetheless, when our intent is to experience life fully, when nothing less than "well-being" is what we're after, then the mirror that intimacy holds up to us shows a challenging and welcome path.

Choosing to care

Emotional awareness is supported and extended by relationship and caring. The more deeply we invest and involve ourselves the more we are apt to trigger intense emotion. The following techniques can help us turn this emotion into self awareness that can greatly enrich our lives.

Sub-personality theory—an aid to the exploration of personality

The most powerful and easy to use concept for extending emotional awareness I know of is based on the assumption that all of us have many aspects to our personalities, some known to us, others unknown. These aspects can be referred to as sub-personalities. The sub-personalities are like the crew of a ship. They have different faces, and they perform different tasks. Some, like the first mate of a ship, are more powerful and active than others, but all have their place and are necessary in order for the ship to move swiftly and safely through the water. The captain is in charge of this crew, and the part of our personality which, like the captain,

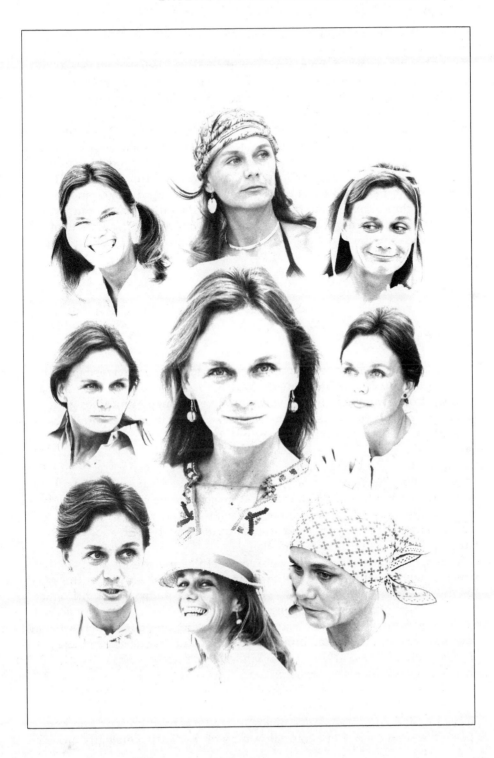

directs the sub-personalities we will name the "ego" simply because ego is a convenient word. The "ego" in this system is conceived of as the core or most basic aspect of the personality, the part we usually call self. It is characterized by feelings of clarity, purposefulness, calm, openness, and receptivity. Ego has the capacity to direct with balanced intention all of he various sub-personalities. Now occasionally the crew or a part of the crew will take over the responsibility of running the ship. When this happens at a personality level we say that a sub-personality—or part—is running the whole—or the "ego." For example, a sub-personality such as the critical part or the child part can take over and run our lives. The theory of sub-personalities and the technique of voice dialogue intends to bring into awareness the roles that sub-personalities play in our lives.[1] By uncovering and clarifying the many and often conflicting aspects of our personality, the ego can take firm hold and provide a balancing aspect in our lives.

Voice dialogue

Voice dialogue is a technique for getting to know ourselves better. It can acquaint us in a nonjudgmental way with aspects of ourselves that are hidden from awareness. In any moment there are many processes going on at the personality level and the choice we make in focusing on only one of these at a time is an arbitrary but useful tool in enhancing self-awareness.

A shift in our energy level and point of view takes place as one or another sub-personality surfaces. For example, I can leave a meeting where I experience myself as bright, calm and insightful, get into my car heading for a destination that is new to me and within a few minutes be close to tears feeling hopelessly lost and stupid. Unfortunately, I do a lot of driving in my "stupid" sub-personality.

Some of the more common sub-personalities include the hurt child, the mother, the father, the hero, the princess, the nebbish ("poor thing," as in "so-and-so, poor thing, can't even . . ."), the dummy, the critic and the punisher. One of my favorites is the demonic, which for many years I associated with all that was "bad" in me including, because I am a woman, my sexuality and desire for influence in the world. *The demonic for many has far more to do with the desire for influence and self-expression than anything inherently evil or immoral.*

As various parts of our personalities emerge and find appropriate expression, we experience ourselves enriched, enlivened, in control of ourselves and energized. Voice dialogue can be carried on with another person or used as part of a journal writing or meditative dialogue process.

EXTENDING EMOTIONAL AWARENESS | 85

Prepare yourself for voice dialogue work by relaxing deeply. (Refer if necessary to techniques for de-stressing that you will find in the section on stress.) Quiet your mind, releasing your usual thought patterns. Focus on that aspect of your personality which we have called "the witness" or impartial observer. (Refer to the witness state in the chapter on "Beginning with Awareness" and see Exercise 1.) The interested, nonjudgmental part simply collects information in a sympathetic, good-natured and often good-humored way. This is the part you will call on in the role of facilitator.

The facilitator's role in voice dialogue

The facilitator's role in voice dialogue is to explore and bring to the attention of the ego various sub-personalities. All sub-personalities are accepted and respected equally—when this is not the case, they won't reveal themselves to us. The facilitator or objective observer is just intending to get to know the personality better, and he/she wants the ego to share in the knowledge of this information, trusting that the value in the process for the moment is simply clarification. In time, this kind of process tends to strengthen our egos. As various parts of our personalities emerge and find appropriate expression, we experience ourselves enriched, enlivened, in control of ourselves and energized.

When you are working by yourself you have to be able to jump back and forth between a facilitating focus and your personality with its ego and sub-personalities.

Another thing to keep in mind is that when you address a sub-personality you are speaking to someone who has moved into an altered state of consciousness. Never leave a sub-personality hanging. To do so can leave a person feeling disoriented and light-headed. Always begin and end by speaking with the ego.

This is a process that takes some uninterrupted time. Don't try to do it in ten minutes. Some sub-personalities—particularly those that are new or have not been active—may take a while to focus in. Don't be in a hurry. And again, suspend judgment and any desire to change a sub-personality. You can bet that when the intention is simply to clarify and bring into focus the sub-personality the appropriateness of its function will emerge eventually.

All sub-personalities are functional

I have worked with many sub-personalities that first came on the scene as villains, critical and self-punishing parts that apparently had no function other that to torment us. In an environment of acceptance, where the facilitator doesn't criticize, judge or punish, the good reasons for the sub-personalities' presence in our lives begin to emerge. The critic, for example, may be trying to protect us from the criticism of others. Sub-personalities are often created when we're very young. What may have seemed protective to a two- or three-year-old may not seem protective to an adult. By uncovering the source of a sub-personality we give it and our egos an opportunity to reevaluate its function and place in our lives.

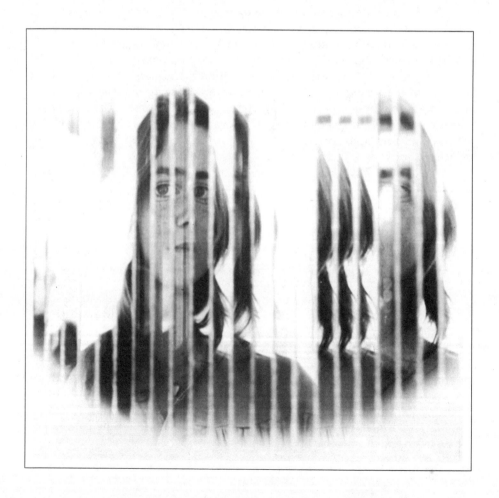

The following will give you an opportunity to experience your sub-personalities.

Exercise 28 — Speaking with Your Sub-Personalities

1. Begin by following the relaxing and focusing suggestions made earlier in this chapter.

2. Concentrate on the facilitating aspect of yourself.

3. Select a sub-personality to engage. A dialogue might begin as follows:

Facilitator to Ego: Hello. How are you today? Is there a particular sub-personality you would like to dialogue with, or would you like me to choose one that I would like to talk with?

Ego: I think I would like to talk to the part of me that eats when I'm full. I would like to get to know that part better.

Facilitator: OK. Shall we call that part the "Overeater"? Overeater, I would like to talk to you.

Overeater: (Overeater moves over, reinforcing the shift from the ego to the sub-personality.)

Facilitator: Hello. How are you today? (Pause to give the sub-personality a chance to focus and collect herself/himself.)

Overeater: Hello. I'm fine.

Facilitator: Tell me about yourself. (Facilitator may use questions such as the following to get the conversation going.) How long have you been around in so-and-so's life? How much time do you take up? Do you like so-and-so? Why? Why do you do what you do? How do you feel? What would you like so-and-so to do? What would you like to tell or say to so-and-so?

4. Begin your own dialogue with a sub-personality.

As you work with sub-personalities, here are some additional points to keep in mind.

A physical move is made each time a new sub-personality is engaged. If, for example, the facilitator asks to speak to the sub-personality "fear," the transition from ego to sub-personality is reinforced by physically moving over to another chair or a new spot in the room. When you write by yourself, a new heading is given every time you address a sub-personality, and when you are dialoguing in meditation, a change in voice, image or smell, etc., is called for.

The facilitator asks reporter-like questions that don't carry judgment.

And of course only one question at a time is asked. A barrage of questions would overwhelm a sub-personality.

The following exercise in writing will further describe sub-personalities.

Exercise 29 — Writing to the Parts of Myself

1. Relax yourself.

2. Ask yourself what sub-personality needs attention or is demanding it, and begin.

3. If you're having trouble starting, the following example might be of help:

Facilitator: Hello, Jeanne (my name), how are you today? Is there a sub-personality that you would like to talk to?

Ego: (Named Jeanne in my case) Hi. Yes, there is. I would like to talk to the part of Jeanne that takes care of her physical body.

Facilitator: Terrific. Let me talk to that part of Jeanne connected with her body. (Pause.) Are you here? (It can be helpful to physically move over at this point.)

The voice of Jeanne's physical body: Yes, I'm here. But I'm not feeling too strong lately. Jeanne hasn't been spending much time listening to me lately. She has been spending hours writing and drinking coffee.

Facilitator: Sounds like you would like her to be doing something else. Is that a correct assumption?

Body voice: You bet. It's been beautiful outside. I would like to see her spending more time walking and running in the fresh air and sunshine. I also wish she would cut down on the coffee drinking.

Facilitator: Sounds like you're very concerned about Jeanne.

Body voice: Yes, I am, and if she doesn't start paying more attention to me, I'm going to give her more headaches so that she will have to stop writing! In fact, I've given her a few already.

Facilitator: That's very interesting. I would like to reconnect with the ego now. Is that OK?

Body voice: Yes.

Facilitator: Ego, are you there? Do you have a reaction to what the body part said?

Ego: I'm here, and I found what the body voice had to say illuminating. I have been getting headaches lately. I even had my eyes checked, and the doctor could find nothing wrong with them. I've never suffered like this before, so until this moment I didn't put together head pain with the fact that I haven't been outside.

4. As you write you will want to switch focus back and forth from facilitator to ego to sub-personality. Actually moving over or changing chairs as you do this will help to accomplish the shift, especially in the beginning.

Voice dialogue can also be used effectively during a meditation.

The following exercise will guide you in this process.

Exercise 30 — Meditating with Sub-Personalities

1. Focus on your body, relaxing those parts that feel tense through deep breathing, imaging, listening to music, stretching, etc. (If you don't know the beginning steps to meditation, review them by referring to the chapter on "Extending Physical Awareness.")

2. Check to see that thoughts too have been relaxed and released.

3. Once you feel de-stressed, sense in some way — hear, touch, see, smell or taste — the facilitator's presence and begin the dialogue. The following is an example of how such a dialogue might go:

Facilitator: Hello, Jeanne. You seem sad today. Could I talk to your sad part?

Ego: (Internally shift the voice or the face to an ego aspect.) The part I'm in touch with isn't so much sad as vulnerable. I could let you talk to that part.

Facilitator: That would be fine. Hello — vulnerable, are you there?

Vulnerable voice: Yes, I'm here, although I don't know why I'm here.

Facilitator: That's OK. You don't have to know. How long have you been around in Jeanne's life?

Vulnerable voice: Oh, I've been around for a long, long time, although she practically never lets anyone know about me.

Facilitator: Really? Why is that?

Vulnerable voice: She doesn't like me and she thinks no one else will either. She also thinks that if others knew about me they would take advantage of her. The tough part of her that she listens to a lot tells her that it's weak to be vulnerable.

Facilitator: Is that true, are you weak?

> *Vulnerable voice:* Not at all. I'm easily affected by what goes on
> around Jeanne, but I'm not swayed to the degree that I have her
> collapsing or immobile. I can steer as straight a course as any
> part of her, even though I'm very sensitive.
>
> *Facilitator:* Well, I would like to speak once more to Jeanne's ego.
> Are you there, Ego? (Pause.)
>
> *Ego:* Yes, I'm back. Boy, I had no idea that vulnerability could be
> strong and senstitive at the same time. That's new information
> to me.
>
> Thus far only one sub-personality at a time has been addressed. It is
> possible to dialogue with more than one. For example, it would have
> been just as reasonable to dialogue with the "tough part of Jeanne" as
> well as the "vulnerable part of Jeanne." The facilitator would simply
> have said "Goodbye" to the vulnerable voice and asked the tough voice
> to come in—perhaps shifting position in order to deepen the focus. There
> are situations in voice dialogue which make themselves known in rather
> rapid succession. In the beginning it's less confusing to stick with one
> or two voices at a time.

When you are working with sub-personalities, questions and observations will occur. Some general remarks may help you to understand what's going on.

1. Sub-personalities emerge appropriately in both masculine and feminine forms.[3] This has to do with belief systems. As a child, did mother or father do the punishing? Chances are that depending on whether it was mother or father, the sub-personality characterized as punishing will have a masculine or feminine tone.

2. There are some sub-personalities that tend to be overly active. They are around controlling what people think, feel and do much of the time. Occasionally, you will encounter a part that is so pervasive as to be in control just about all of the time. Sub-personalities that tend to be overly active are the critic or faultfinder, the pusher or its opposite, the rebel, the mother in women, and anger or laziness in teenagers. (Voice dialogue is effective with older children and teenagers.) The point again is not to judge or try to manipulate or change the overly active sub-personality. The purpose is to understand how it controls and why it feels the need to be in charge so much of the time.

3. Some sub-personalities are underactive or mute. They may be a part of the personality that never speaks out. Examples include the vulnerable voice, the child voice, and for many people who suffer from dis-ease, the demonic voice.

The "demonic" in our culture is characterized by power in connection with money, sex and assertiveness in the world. People disown the demonic in one form or another because they feel this aspect of themselves to be bad, immoral or unpopular. When this sub-personality is uncritically supported and allowed to emerge, a great deal of energy is often released and available to be used appropriately by the ego.

Disowned or underactive sub-personalities often require a particularly supportive climate in order to speak out. Here is where working with another person who understands and supports the process is especially helpful.

As voice dialogue is engaged in by oneself or in connection with others, the breadth, depth, fullness of human personality comes to light. I personally marvel at the richness and complexity of inner drives and intentions. There is so much to us—so much to be known if we can but give ourselves permission to know it!

Personal journal work

If you have been following the exercises in this book, you are by now familiar with the habit of taking written notes about yourself. Tedious as these may seem at times, the process locks into memory the insights we are gaining about ourselves.[5] This note-taking process can now be expanded into an ongoing dialogue with the most fundamental aspects of your personality. These are the parts of ourselves that we often have the least understanding of, but are the most influential in determining the quality of life we experience. In the preceding section the written exercises with voice dialogue followed the format of a personal journal or diary. The personal journal extends the possibility of self-discovery in a written process. The idea is to think of your notebook as a highly facilitating friend, a very wise and compassionate confidante that is always available at a moment's notice.[6] This friend or buddy is never comparative, judgmental, uninterested or at a loss for words. Moreover, this sensational friend is both masculine and feminine so that sometimes the discussion is with a man and at other times it's with a woman, depending on your need and desire. All this wonderful person asks from us is respect and contact. In order to be the most help to you, the writing will require focus at a time and place that permits your undivided attention.

There are dozens of variations possible with journal writing. You can address any one of your sub-personalities (refer to section on sub-personalities), your higher mind or the God within and without. You can use the journal for all or any of the following purposes:

- To get to know yourself better.
- To see yourself as others see you.
- To reflect on a difficult problem or situation.
- To find creative solutions.
- To find comfort, guidance and inspiration.

The following are brief examples that will give you an idea of some of the possibilities available in journal writing:

1. *Me:* Dear Controller, I would like to understand you better.
   Controller: I'm glad to hear that. I would like you to understand me better too. Maybe then you wouldn't feel so rotten about me.
   Me: Tell me, why do you act the way you do, controlling and manipulating your loved ones?
   Controller: I don't know. I just have this urge — this feeling of tightness in my throat and stomach. It's hard for me to feel relaxed when someone I care about is acting without considering my feelings.
   Me: Do you really expect people to put your feelings before their own consistently?
   Controller: I guess I do. I feel unloved when they don't.
   Me: Is that a very loving attitude on your part?
   Controller: Not really, but I seem to be so unsure about myself that I'm always needing reassurance.

2. *Me:* Dear Creative Part. Boy, do I need your help. I have a paper that's due Monday and I just can't get a handle on what it is I want to say or how I want to say it!
   Creative part: Take it easy! Relaxing will make things easier for you. One thing you could do is to call on me earlier in the future. One day isn't enough time for me to come up with my best effort. However, I'll give it a try.
   Me: Thanks. I'll take a few deep breaths.

The last example is one of communication with your God-like self — your higher mind — that part of you which represents your wisest, most knowing aspects. This is an inner friend that you can turn to for spiritual guidance, understanding and inspiration — the part that is capable of seeing beyond the immediacy of the most difficult moment. This part of you truly understands not only your position and your good reasons for being and doing, but the good reasons behind the behavior of others as well. Compassion and extended knowing characterize this aspect.

3. *Me:* Dear Higher Mind. Life is moving so rapidly for me these days I feel overwhelmed.

Higher mind: Are you unhappy?

Me: No—I like it, but I'm so unsettled inside. I feel out of control.

Higher mind: It just seems that way because you're not used to moving so fast. You're like a toddler learning to walk who is used to crawling. There will be stumbles and maybe a bumped nose, but you'll get up and grow.

Me: And my fears about falling and really getting hurt—what do I do with them?

Higher mind: Let it be part of your awareness as you experience yourself in new ways. Let it be and you will be alright.

Remember to keep in mind as you do the journal work that the purpose of this process is clarity, self-understanding and awareness. Take time, probe a little and get to know well this person that you are. When you hold back judgment and comparison you're much more apt to succeed in this intention. *Detachment from urgency is the key to gaining a fresh perspective.* The aspect of yourself that you address—inner friend, creative part, etc.—has clarity precisely because it's not attached or invested in the problem. That part is always more interested in you and your well-being process than in a specific problem, and that's precisely why problem solving in this way can be so effective.

The following exercise will give you greater familiarity with the personal journal process.

Exercise 31 — Making Friends with the Friend Within

1. Select a notebook, pencil and pen that please you. Bring awareness into your choice and select the colors, shapes and sizes that appeal to you.

2. Put aside a period of uninterrupted time. You will need at least thirty minutes for this purpose at first. Later the process can take place in less time. When you wake up or just before you go to sleep are especially good times to write.

3. Now begin the written dialogue with your new friend by introducing yourself as you would to someone you trusted immediately. For example, you might begin as follows:

Me: Dear Friend (you might want to give your new friend a name), I'm glad we met and I would like to begin our friendship by telling you all about myself. That includes the things I normally tell new acquaintances about me and the things I might tell, but don't. I am thirty-nine, a good age that makes me old enough to have learned I have choice about whether or not to enjoy my life. I can love and I am loved. I can be myself and I can let others be themselves—usually! I have three children that I'm grateful for, a husband who is my friend, and purposeful work. I'm intense and easily affected. Those are the basics.

Inner friend: You've told me quite a bit, but I'm interested in knowing whether you've left out anything important simply because it's difficult to say.

Me: Well, I suppose I should tell you that I'm a more serious and forceful person than I initially appear to be. You see I don't feel comfortable behaving forcefully in public. I want to be liked and I tend to be protective and this gets in the way of clarity and forcefulness. I'm hoping that writing to you will help me gain awareness of my process in this regard.

Inner friend: Indeed it will. (etc., etc., etc.)

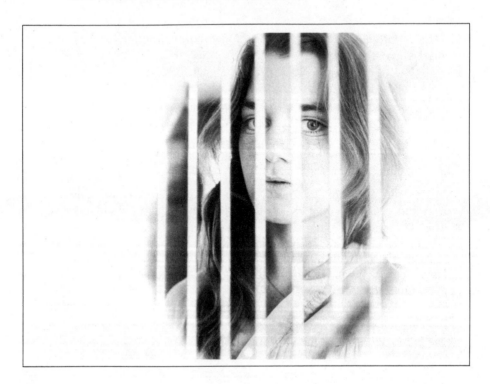

4. Be sure to maintain the dialogue. Don't forget to pause and give the inner friend a chance to acknowledge and respond to what you have said.

5. Your inner friend will speak to you through your body and your *unfocused* mind.

    a. Tune in to your body (refer to Exercise 1 for suggestions on listening to the body) and its inner dialogue—the places of feeling within. This is the voice of your friend speaking to you.

    b. Remember, let go any judgments you may have about the process or the voices within you.

    c. Let the thoughts and words tumble out randomly—don't try to structure or control them.

6. Dialogue like this at least once a day for at least two or three weeks or until it's no longer an effort to do so. After a week or so you will find it much easier to get a fluid and spontaneous dialogue going.

It bears repeating to say that all personal journal work will be deepened by initiating it in a calm and relaxed state. Most people are relaxed in the morning when they awaken and this is therefore an especially good time to write. If you need help and guidance at a time when you are stressed, then take time before you begin to breathe deeply (refer to deep breathing exercise) and relax your body (refer to de-stressing exercises). Sometimes exercise or a brisk walk is helpful in this regard. Eating is usually counterproductive. The less you eat, the more alert your inner friend is apt to be. But don't make this an inflexible rule—just be sure to listen to your body, and avoid "drowning out" the voice of one need by rushing in with food for another.

Remember that this is work you do with an inner self that likes you. Comparisons, judgments, demands and urgency are never a part of this process.

Moving from safety to awareness with others

Sex, togetherness, support and caring or nurturing come to mind when the subject of intimacy and relationship is broached in our culture.[8] Rarely will people think of relationship in connection with self-knowledge, and yet the most amazing self-discoveries occur when our desire is to know and accept without qualification or judgment another human being.

We may discover, for example, capacities for strength, tenderness, understanding and wisdom that we never dreamed were contained within us.

Much of the time beyond courtship, change rather than knowledge or understanding is the focus of our intent. We have in mind the way we want intimates to be, the way intimates "should" be in order to measure up to our expectations and we want them to change. We want them to be other than what they are. Generally, the last thing we want when we're feeling uncomfortable or when we're wanting is to understand how the other feels. Judgment, blame and the desire to alter someone's behavior overcome our interest in knowing and understanding. It's relatively easy to trust someone, to have faith in their goodwill, to be sincerely interested —until the other's behavior provokes discomfort in us. It's so much easier to say they're wrong than to question the appropriateness of our own response.

Next time you have a disagreement with someone important to you, call in the impartial observer and ask, *"What is most important to me in this moment—understanding and clarification, or getting the other to be different?"* Do you really want to understand why your kid won't clean up his room, or why your mate is not interested in you, or why your mother insists on telling you what to do? When the answer is "yes," sooner or later you will understand and most likely learn a thing or two about yourself in the process. For example, when I asked my teenage son to share his reasons for not straightening his room, he led me to understand that tidiness, as the result of pressure from me, diminished self-respect in his eyes. When he said "no" to me, he felt a measure of independence that made him like himself better. By wanting to know rather than blame or insist, I learned two important things, one about him and the other about me. The first was that what the boy was making was a choice to feel good—not to hurt me. The second was that I was pressuring him to change. Most of the time, however, when we observe ourselves and answer the question honestly and without self-judgment, it will be "no." "No—what I want is for them to be different now!" To be aware of ourselves in this context and to turn the question around to oneself, asking "Why don't I want to know them?" or "Why do I want to change them?" constitutes a leap in psychological awareness. Working with these questions in journal dialogue (refer to the section on voice dialogue) or bringing them into meditation can be an illuminating exercise.

The teacher who bites

When an area in our body becomes quite tense in situations with others that are clearly *not* life-threatening, then often what's going on is that a little salt is being rubbed into our beliefs about who we are.

We have at such times come face to face with a suddenly triggered disowned sub-personality. For example, a singularly meek man or woman may burn inside when confronted with the presence of an assertive or aggressive individual. The reverse can also be true—a singularly aggressive person can become very upset and uncertain in the presence of someone who is very timid.

At other times, the situation triggers the negativity we feel in regard to a part of ourselves that we *do* have some knowledge of, but haven't fully accepted and integrated in our lives. Self-centered and self-indulgent individuals, for example, evoked "gut level anger" in me until I acknowledged and made peace with the depth of my own selfishness. Now when I am with singularly self-involved people, I see the limitation, but it doesn't touch me in a negative way. I know that I too am self-centered, but not exclusively so and not in a way that limits the quality of life for myself and others. I may not choose to spend much time with someone who is consistently self-engrossed and not interested in me or anyone else, but my stomach no longer clutches in their presence.

I am not saying that life does not confront us with people and situations that we simply don't like. There is much to be seen that is frustrating, disheartening and sad. Nonetheless, *when we have freed ourselves from singularly emotional response inflicted by "the teacher," we are in a better position to constructively affect any situation we find ourselves in.*

The following exercises will help you to understand your own motivations better.

Exercise 32 — Using a Personal Journal to Illuminate Relationship

In your personal journal have your "facilitator" address the following questions to you during a period when you are feeling unhappy with your child, parent, mate, boss, friend, etc.:

1. What do I expect from _____?
2. Do I really want to understand _____'s motivation?
3. Do I really want to know _____? If the answer is "no," then ask, "Why don't I really want to know them?"
4. Do I want to change them more than I want to know them? If the answer to this question is "yes," then ask yourself, "Why do I want to change them?"

5. Remember that the facilitator is a nonjudgmental, friendly observer. However you spontaneously answer these questions, it's OK. You are collecting information about yourself that can ultimately enhance the quality of your life. Set aside judgments, comparisons and expectations in order to learn. (See Brugh Joy, *Joy's Way.*)

6. If you have answered the above questions "No, I don't want to know or understand," just hold this awareness and ask yourself the following question: How do I feel when I'm around people who want to change me?

7. Continue to observe yourself in this way over the next two or three months.

Exercise 33 — Using Meditation to Illuminate Relationship

1. Take a few deep breaths. Relax yourself deeply, letting go your usual thoughts and concerns.

2. Follow whatever practice you normally would in initiating meditation: deep breathing, concentration, listening to music, etc.

3. At the point where you feel yourself shift into a more deeply relaxed state than when you began, begin a dialogue between yourself and your witness or facilitator. Have your facilitator ask the following questions:

    a. Do you (ego) really want to know and understand _____?

    b. If the answer is "no." ask, "Why don't I want to understand _____?"

    c. Do I want to change _____?

    d. If the answer is "yes," ask, "Why do I want to change _____?"

You can also address questions about relationship when you're not troubled or unhappy with a particular relationship. However, as I said earlier, when people are behaving in ways that we like, we don't feel threatened and are apt to respond ourselves in customary ways. There is therefore less likelihood that we will learn something new about ourselves. Another very helpful way of exploring in regard to relationship is by doing voice dialogue work together (refer to section on voice dialogue).

Very often there are sub-personalities at work in our relationships that require this process in order to be fully revealed. The facilitator might speak to the angry part or the withdrawn part, etc., in order to bring understanding and clarity to the situation. The following is an example of a dyadic process ("dyad" means "pair") where the intent is to know rather than to assign blame or to make judgments about right and wrong.

> *Facilitator:* Hello, I would like to speak to the icy, withdrawn part. (No judgment is made that might suggest there is something bad or wrong with the icy, withdrawn part. All sub-personalities are treated cordially.)
>
> *Icy, withdrawn part:* The person being addressed moves over to signify a shift from the ego to the sub-personality.) Hello. (Pause.) What do you want?
>
> *Facilitator:* I would like some clarification about who you are and the role you play in _____'s life.
>
> *Icy-withdrawn:* I protect her. I keep her from getting hurt. I protect her by punishing others when they hurt or disappoint her.
>
> *Facilitator:* How do you do that?
>
> *Icy-withdrawn:* I don't speak to them, and I act like I don't like them.
>
> *Facilitator:* How does that protect _____?
>
> *Icy-withdrawn:* Well, usually I get activated when _____ has been hurt. By withdrawing I protect _____ from getting hurt even more. (etc., etc.)

Wanting to know rather than to change a person is half the picture when it comes to intimacy and relationship. The other half is the willingness to allow oneself to be fully known and to let another see the effect they have on us.

I have never experienced a person who did not want to be known, although I have experienced many who were afraid to be known.

The value in revealing oneself lies in the wonderful feeling of self-acceptance and surge of energy that is connected to being exactly who we are. It is also true that we can never fully experience ourselves being loved and accepted by others until we are willing to share fully with them.

If it is true that intimacy has so much value attached to it—and it does—then why are people so reluctant to involve themselves in it?

The answer is fear. The following are some of the more common fears people associate with intimacy:

1. Fear of losing oneself—of giving up personal identity in exchange for being loved.

2. Fear of not being lovable, acceptable or good, or good enough.

3. Fear of loss of control, not being in charge of myself and/or my life.

4. Fear of rejection and abandonment, of not being liked, accepted or loved.

Whatever we're afraid of, two things are likely to be true:

1. *Fear is not likely to be expressed directly as fear, but rather through manipulating and controlling behaviors toward ourselves and others.*

2. *The patterns of fear—manipulation and control—arose as the result of the interaction we perceived with our parents in early childhood.* The way we related with intimates then is the way we're apt to relate today.

Awareness is again the key that gives us the possibility of moving beyond these patterns into new ones that extend well-being.

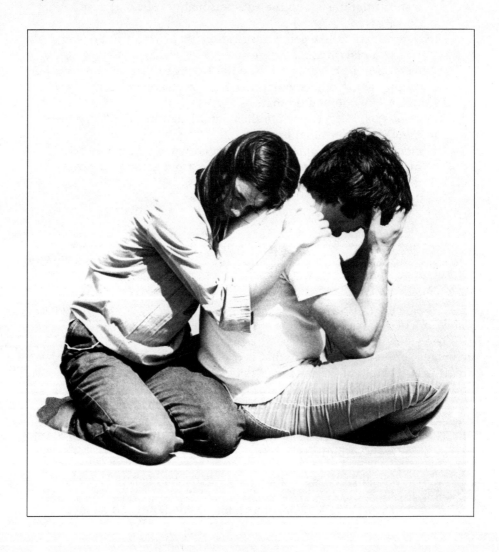

The following exercise can extend awareness of fear in regard to intimacy and relationship with others.

Exercise 34 — Tuning into Fear of Intimacy

1. Make the following resolution by writing it down or taking it into meditation. (Refer to Exercise 31 and Exercise 32 on personal journal work.) The next time I find myself more than momentarily upset with someone important to me, I will ask myself the following question: "What part or parts of my body are tense — tight or heavy — in this moment of distress?"

2. Ask yourself, "Do I feel the feelings that I associate with fear?" If the answer from your body is in any way "yes," then continue by asking, "What am I afraid of?" Possibilities might include rejection, abandonment, feelings of inadequacy, loss of control, loss of self.

3. Tune into the physical feelings and ask, "When in the past do I remember feeling this way?" Let the memories progressively take you back to earlier and earlier periods in your life.

4. If it is possible for you to take a few minutes off in the moment, reflect on the above in your personal journal or in meditation. (Refer to Exercise 32 on the personal journal and Exercise 33 on meditation.)

The experiences we fear are those we associate with pain, and for many if not all a correlation exists between early experiences with intimates and emotional pain. Memories include hurtful feelings of rejection, abandonment, inadequacy and loss of personal identity.

In addition to emotional pain, there are hurtful early memories for many that include poverty, hunger, disease, physical abuse and deprivation.

All or any of these memories can lead to patterns of fear and manipulation in present-day relationships.

While avoidance of pain may be the intention behind much stressful interaction, what is expressed most of the time are strategies of manipulation that attempt to avoid the pain. Rather than face the awareness of our hurt and our fear of hurt, we control to avoid it by manipulating ourselves and others. Common patterns directed toward intimates include threatening with anger, guilt, shame, punishment and withdrawal of love. Patterns for self-manipulation include denial of that which we feel, including fear and hurt.

The following exercise will help bring manipulating patterns to awareness. It can be done with another person, by yourself in meditation or through personal journal work. (Refer to Exercise 32 on the personal journal and Exercise 30 on Meditating with Sub-Personalities.)

Exercise 35 — Meeting the Relationship Manipulator

1. Initiate a dialogue with that sub-personality we will call the relationship manipulator.

    a. The dialogue might begin as follows:

      Facilitator to Ego: I would like to speak with the part of your personality that manipulates in intimate relationships.

      Ego: OK.

      Relationship manipulator: (Moves over to indicate shift to sub-personality.) Hello.

      Facilitator: I'm glad to meet you. Tell me, how do you operate in intimate relationships? (etc., etc.)

    b. The facilitator might go on to ask how active this part is or how much energy is invested in manipulating behaviors. Other illuminating questions might include: How long have you been active? Do you manipulate in the same ways with everyone, or are you more active with some people than others? What would happen if you manipulated less?

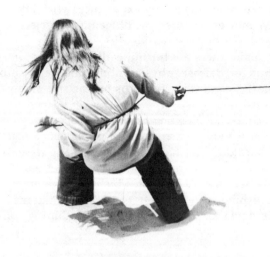

> 2. Keep in mind that the intention of the dialogue is to collect infor-
> mation and expand awareness. Suspend judgment and don't worry about
> understanding all that may be revealed.

Pain isn't necessarily an enemy

Many of us have experienced a debilitating sense of helplessness connected with feelings of sadness and hurt when we were children. Youngsters are not in a position to understand or move away from people and situations they find hurtful. As adults, we have choice, and within the context of choice, sadness and pain are experiences we can do something about. Painful feelings can guide us toward a more rewarding and fulfilling life. They teach us what not to do and they can also teach us about ourselves. In situations, for example, where we feel badly for no apparent reason we can ask why and follow the feelings to the source within us.

The function of pain is to enable healing to take place. When we allow ourselves to consciously feel deeply sad, we promote the mending of old wounds and the release of energy that results in extended intelligence, creativity and physical energy. Moreover, we bring into being a youthful capacity for experiencing life joyously. As adults we have the opportunity to live our lives with the intensity of a child, balanced by experience and choice based on awareness.

With awareness comes choice. As we continue to bring focus and clarity into our intimate relationships, possibilities for change present themselves. When we feel afraid and we know it, we can manipulate ourselves by denial or the behavior of others through various controls, or we can stay with the experience of our feelings. This direct experience of ourselves may include real pain as well as the fear of pain. A loved one may not choose to do that which pleases us. When this is the case, we may feel sadness and disappointment, and these are certainly not longed-for experiences. However, some measure of sadness and disappointment in a close relationship is unavoidable, especially when we are accepting of the other's individuality and not intent on changing them. Another way of saying this is that when we truly love and honor others we will not always be pleased ourselves. However, if our intention is to love rather than to change, and to know and be ourselves fully, then we will be willing to experience a measure of sadness and disappointment. The rewards will be sufficiently great to get us through the difficult periods, for with love in our lives the quality of life and well-being is enhanced immeasurably.

Awareness makes love and relationship wonder full

Awareness extends our capacity to truly hear and experience ourselves and others without shutting out, spacing out, or becoming defensive. Love happens when we listen with the intention of fully hearing. In order to listen to others in this way, we must explore and understand our own needs. Satisfaction or resolution may result from awareness of what it is we want. However, it is not necessary to resolve neediness in order to love, as long as these needs are out in the open. As you experienced this chapter, insights may have emerged that conflicted with some of your basic beliefs about how you or those important to you ought to be or act. If your intention is to "right those wrongs" and you don't really have the power to do this you will tend to block or inhibit your awareness. If however, you believe that awareness is valuable because it leads to a deeper knowing and consequent loving of oneself and other, then you will experience even painful awareness as an opportunity for a richer and fuller life.

Notes to Chapter IV

[1]Voice dialogue technique was first introduced to me by Dr. Harold Stone (see H. Stone and S. Winkelman, "Voice Dialogue: A Tool for Transformation"). It is a preferred technique of the Research Clinic at the Center for the Healing Arts in Los Angeles. In my work I have modified the technique to serve my purposes and intentions.

[2]Dr. F. Perls (see *In and Out the Garbage Pail* and *Gestalt Therapy Verbatim*) first suggested changing chairs to reflect differing parts of the personality.

[3]C. G. Jung (see *Memories, Dreams, Reflections*) first introduced the concept of archetypical male and female personalities such as the "hero" or the "mother" that are universally shared.

[4]Dr. B. Joy (see *Joy's Way*) introduced me to the concept of "discernment."

[5]See I. Progoff, *At a Journal Workshop: The Basic Text and Guide for Using the Intensive Journal.*

[6]See A. Nin, *The Diary of Anais Nin, 1931–1934*; F. Perls, *In and Out the Garbage Pail*; B. Stevens, *Don't Push the River.*

[7]See E. Fromm, *The Art of Loving;* M. and J. Paul, *Free to Love;* C. R. Rogers, *On Becoming a Person;* V. Satir, *Peoplemaking.*

[8]Many of the concepts and ideas presented here regarding intimacy and relationship have been explored creatively by Jordan and Margaret Paul, close friends for over twenty years. Their forthcoming book is titled *Do I Have To Give Myself Up In Order To Be Loved By You?*, published by J. P. Tarcher.

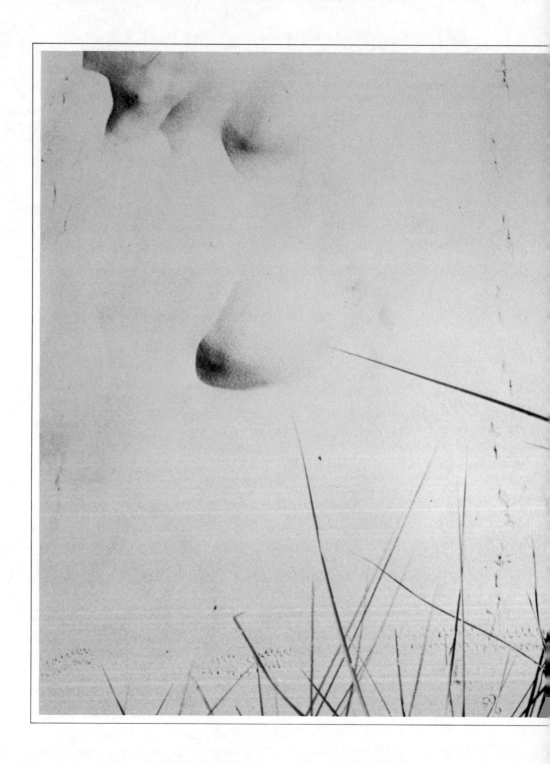

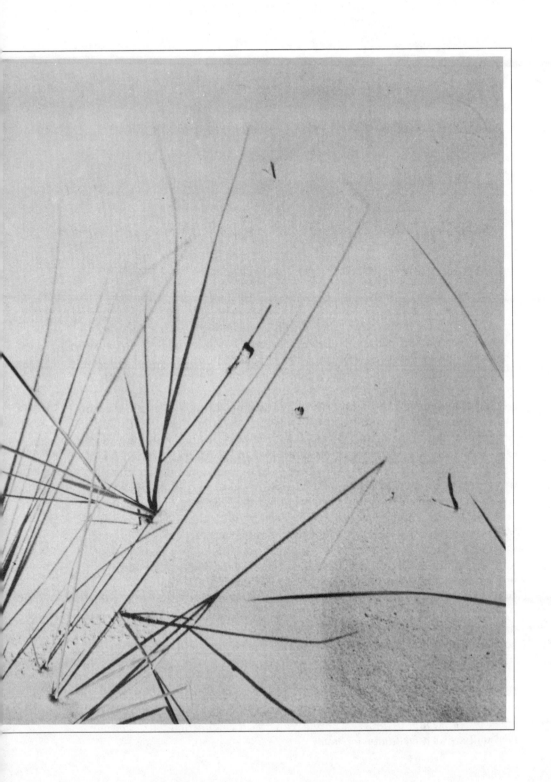

5

Extending Your Mental Capacities

Your brain belongs to you. It's yours to do with as you will—
yours to feed, to stretch, to explore, to expand and above all to use in ways
that will extend the quality of life for yourself and others. Your brain is the
single most powerful and direct connection you have with well-being. It
controls every cell in your physical body, and therefore the ways you
perceive, feel, experience and create. In addition, as part of a mind-brain
system, it may be your link with the universe and immortality. This last
function of the brain is not as yet scientifically verifiable, although there
is a growing body of evidence collected that links our minds with a universal system.[1] This system is suggestive of a hologram.[2] A hologram is
a picture, the smallest part of which contains a rough outline of the original in its entirety. Holograms do exist, and the theory proposed suggests
that our brains could be part of such a system with universal connections.
Vast amounts of information could be contained within our brains in a
form less clear and direct than we are used to. This theory is, of course,
still speculative. What is not speculative is the fact that we apparently
engage only about five percent of our brain most of the time. The question. I find tremendously exciting are: Can we learn to tap into the other
ninety-five percent, and if so, how? Personal experience, not involving
drug use, has led me to believe that all people can consciously gain
access to more and more of their brains. This section will suggest attitudes and exercises for facilitating this process.

*Since intelligence is what most people will first think of in connection with
the brain, the following exercise explores the way we conceive of ourselves
intellectually. The questions can be asked in written form in your journal, or
taken into a meditative process, or worked with in conjunction with someone
who will act as a facilitator for you.*

Exercise 36 — Questions about My Intelligence

1. Do I really believe that I'm intelligent? How would I rate my intelligence?

2. Does my brain function for me? Can I count on my mind to help me get out of puzzling and difficult situations?

3. Do I trust my mind—my perceptions, my impressions—or do I let others tell me how and what to think?

4. Do I value intelligence—is it an asset or a liability?

5. Does doing something dumb make me dumb?

6. When I use my head to solve a problem is it a pleasurable experience for me?

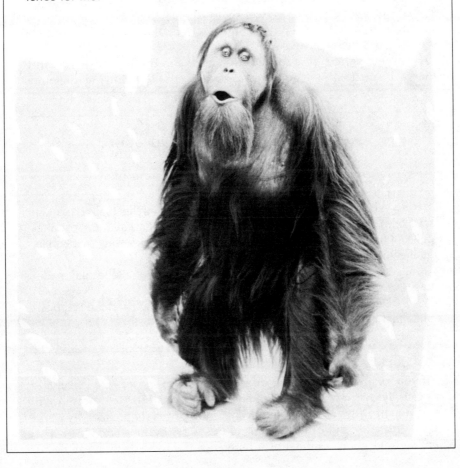

What do you come up with? Are you satisfied with yourself intellectually, are you bright enough, too bright, or less than what you would wish to be? In the fifties, when I was a high school student, it was unpopular to be too bright—especially if you were a girl, and many wishing to be "in" and "attractive" disowned their intelligence.[3]

Disowning intelligence

There are many ways we have of disowning intelligence. It's often disowned when it's not understood or appreciated by those we look up to or have looked up to. It's disowned in processes where we tell ourselves we are stupid or inadequate; it's disowned in belief systems that view intelligence as something unchangeable and fixed like the color of our eyes, instead of a very fluid system that can vary greatly and is influenced by all kinds of factors, including diet, exercise, emotional well-being and, above all, one's belief systems.

If you're a person who for one reason or another has disowned intelligence, go back to a dialoguing process and ask the following questions:

Exercise 37 — Follow-up Questions about Intelligence

1. Have I always felt inadequate intellectually?

2. When did I first begin to feel inadequate intellectually? You can start from a more recent memory and move back, asking after each recalled situation: "And before that, when do I recall feeling inadequate intellectually?"

3. What do I do to myself to maintain a sense of intellectual inadequacy?

4. Do I really want to fully own my intelligence and the responsibility that may be connected with this ownership?

If you hesitated on the last question in the exercise, "Do I really want to fully own my intelligence and the responsibility connected with this ownership?" you're not alone. There are probably as many rewards for being dumb and "out of it" in this culture as for being smart, or so it seems when we hold up as a model of intelligence the hard-driving intellectual or professional. The thing to keep in mind is that within a perspective that values well-being and views it as a lifelong process, intelligence and the full use of all one's mental capacities is part of a lifestyle that is balanced by attention also given to the body, the emotions and the spirit.

The first step, therefore, in reclaiming or expanding intelligence is to choose to like and use your brain—to conceive of it as friend and support to well-being. This friend can be a dependable source for guidance, problem-solving, inspiration, comfort and healing once you're consciously connected to these possibilities.

A very brief and simple description of the brain will give you an idea of why so much is possible. The brain mass that fills the top of the skull is largely made up of two great hemispheres—the left and the right. Each hemisphere has its own functions to perform in relation to the body, and each is capable of functioning independently of the other. The two are connected, however, through an intermediary area called the corpus callosum. Substantially more is known about the left hemisphere, which controls the right half of the body, than the right, which controls the left. The left side houses those centers that control conscious mental functioning. When we recall, speak and think deductively, we do so from the left hemisphere of our brains. The right hemisphere houses the centers for that part of experience we label unconscious—those that become activated when we dream, fantasize, create, intuit and sense. This very large part of the brain is relatively unknown, but a very real possibility exists today for gaining conscious access to this enormously rich source of intellectual experience and knowing. Moreover, since every cell in our body is connected to our brain, *as we gain access to more of our mental capacity, the possibility for consciously controlling physical functioning that was thought to be beyond intentional control does exist.* Another exciting possibility has to do with conscious use of several mental processes simultaneously, that is, thinking and perceiving several different things in any one moment. All of this points to possibilities for using our minds more fully to enhance the quality of life for ourselves and others.

Disinhibiting the brain

Once you've decided to allow yourself to stretch and expand your brain, the first step is to loosen or disinhibit the fixed patterns within which you function much of the time mentally.

The following exercises offer a variety of ways in which to disrupt the linear verbal patterns that many are locked into. The first of these takes you back to an experience of language during a time in life when your brain was growing at an accelerated rate.

Exercise 38 — Disinhibiting with Make-Believe Language

1. Imagine that you're very young and pretend to speak a foreign language out loud. It of course comes out as gobbledegook. You may find that your gobbledegook sounds like several foreign languages all mixed up together. Go ahead, that's terrific!
2. Don't try to figure out what you are saying; pay attention to what you feel and let the nonsense sounds tumble out accordingly.
3. Don't be afraid to raise and lower your voice.
4. Imagine that you're having an argument, being persuasive, making love, etc., in your special language.
5. Keep dialoguing with the nonsense sounds for two or three minutes *out loud.*

This is a wonderful exercise to do when you're mentally stuck. I advise it daily as a kind of mental calisthenic. Since it only takes a few minutes of privacy, you can do it during short car trips, when you're alone in an elevator, in the shower, etc.

Another method for interrupting routine mental patterns with a novel practice incorporates music with problem solving.

Exercise 39 — Disinhibiting with Sound[4]

1. Select a problem in your life that you're having a hard time with.
2. Choose a piece of music or a sound pattern, such as the sea, to listen to that fully involves you.
3. Lie down, take a few deep breaths and deeply relax yourself. (Refer to sections on deep breathing and de-stressing.)
4. If it's music you're listening to, turning up the volume may involve you more. Surrender to the sound — melt into it.

5. Now bring your problem back into focus and give it to the music or sound to solve.
   a. Let images and feelings flash before you.
   b. Don't try to control what's happening. Stay with the sound and whatever flashes of insight, words, sounds, pictures, smells, tastes, etc., that come to you.
6. Write your experience down in your journal. (Refer to suggestions on using the personal journal.)

The following exercise will extend and enhance the process of self-observation as well as calm you before sleeping.

Exercise 40 — Disinhibiting the Experiences of the Day before Sleep[4]

1. From the objective position of a dispassionate observer, review the happenings of the day.
   a. In your cataloguing move from those events that took place at the end of the day toward those that took place at the beginning.
   b. The trick here is to conduct this review without judgments one way or the other. Those events that you put in good or bad categories, that hurt or angered you or elated you, are experienced this time around simply as happenings. Everything that you experienced is interpreted as a lesson. Life is teaching you what to do and what not to do.
2. Don't be surprised to find yourself falling asleep before you have completed your list of the day's activities. That's fine. It's the process, not its length, that's important. Your sleep will be deep and very restful.

It is appropriate to mention meditation again — here as a disinhibiting agent for routine mental processes. It is pleasant to know that when we clear and quiet our minds we may be promoting increased mental functioning even as we de-stress and relax.

Another way to disengage the usual mental patterns is by pairing them with something out of the ordinary.

The following exercise connects a thinking process to an object in nature.

Exercise 41—Disinhibiting Using Objects in Nature to Reveal the Patterning of Our Lives[4]

1. Go outside and carefully select a rock, a piece of bark, a leaf, shell, etc., that intrigues you.

2. Find a comfortable, quiet place and spend some time just looking intently at the patterning you observe in the natural form you have selected to gaze at.

3. Now ask yourself the following question: "How does this patterning reveal patterns in my own life? What does it teach me about myself and conditions in my life?"

4. You might want to dialogue with the leaf, stone, shell, etc., to gain deeper insight. (Refer to dialoguing techniques under "Personal Journal Work.")

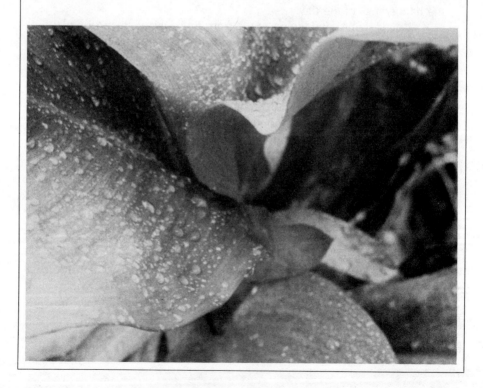

The most difficult mental patterns to break are those to which we attach a lot of feeling. If you have been stretching your capacity to view yourself as an impartial observer (refer to the suggestions on expanding awareness in the "Beginning with Awareness" chapter), you already have a valuable tool for disinhibiting unwanted thoughts. To observe oneself with clarity and detachment is in itself an interruption of the usual.

Expanding perception

All the information processed by your brain is perceived first by one or more of your senses. In order to have consciousness of something you must first see, hear, touch, smell or taste it. I believe there is at least one more sense—an intuitive sense which probably brings in information through the body's energy fields. In other words, your intellect learns about life through your senses. The more sensitive and developed these senses are, the more information they carry and the more clearly we perceive "what's out there."

The following exercise, taken directly from the work of Robert Masters and Jean Houston, will help to extend the quality and range of your senses.

Exercise 42—Clearing and Cleaning the Rooms of Perception

1. Begin by taking a few deep breaths and deeply relaxing yourself. (Refer to Exercise 21 on deep breathing.)

2. Imagine yourself walking up the stairs of a grand old house. You open the door and go in. The first door you see is labeled the "Room of Light." This room represents your visual sense. You open the door and step inside to a room that looks like it has not been cleaned in years. It could be magnificent, but it's a mess! Look around, really see the room, touch parts of it, smell it, listen as you move through it, sense it in every way that you can. Now begin to clean up the mess. Feel yourself washing, dusting, polishing and see the room that represents your visual sense begin to take shape and shine! Now stand back and admire your handiwork. Feel your vision cleared and extended. See yourself seeing more and better!

---

3. At this point you notice a door at the back labeled the "Room of Sound" leading to yet another totally different room. You open it and again you discover a messy, dusty room, this time representing your auditory sense. It too has the potential for being magnificent. Set to work as you did initially, really feeling, seeing, hearing, smelling and if possible tasting the space, and your experience of clearing and cleaning it. Experience yourself hearing more acutely. As you stand back admiring your handiwork, you notice yet another door at the back of this room.

4. You approach next a door labeled the "Room of Smell," and again you find yourself in an entirely different space that once more looks like it hasn't been cleaned for years. Repeating the above process, you move next to the "Room of Taste," then the "Room of Touch."

5. The final room you visit is larger than all the rest combined, and the door leading to it names it the "Room of Intuition." For the final time you find yourself in a gigantic and entirely new room. Look it over, carefully noticing every detail and involving yourself as fully as possible in the process of restoring it. When you're finished, experience the extension of your intuitive sense.

6. The entire exercise usually takes from five to fifteen minutes. Try doing it once a week to stimulate and sharpen your sensory awareness.

Exercise 42 is an example of how you can use imagined experiences to influence and affect mental processes. The power of engaging your imagination to affect mental processes is underscored by the fact that *all information carried to the brain is recorded,* although not necessarily available to memory, including imagined sensory experiences. *Our belief systems, our feelings about ourselves and others, and our behavior are based on the sum total of perceived information, both real and imagined.* This affords us the opportunity to positively affect our own beliefs, feelings and behavior by conveying appropriate imagined sensory impressions to the brain. In this way, with mental pictures, we can actually teach our brains and shape our consciousness.

Extending mental processes through movement

Research and observation point out the correlation between physical and mental activity. Periods of greatest mental growth in life correspond to those times when we have been physically active and moved in a great variety of ways. Brain research suggests that the reason toddlers around three years of age learn so much so fast has to do with the spontaneous and inventive way in which they move. Go to a park and take a good look at the three-year-olds playing. Observe that they never seem to make the same movement twice in a row, and while you do this keep in mind that they're learning every second! Research with the aged backs this correlation up, for amazing changes have taken place, including apparent reversal of senility, when a variety of movements become daily practice for the elderly. (Refer to the Feldenkrais work with the aged that is discussed earlier in this book in the section "Learning to Move.") Movement that varies is therefore an important factor in enhancing and extending mental activity.

The following is a physical exercise that you will find clears your mind, awakens and refreshes you mentally. Try it when you're tired and observe how reviving it can be.

Exercise 43 — Moving as if You Were Three Years Old[4]

1. If you don't have a three-year-old handy, go to a park and observe the movement patterns of toddlers. Notice that they not only walk forward but backward and sideways as well. Notice also that they quickly change vertical positions. Within a few seconds they may stand, sit, roll, squat or lie down.

2. Now go home and do what you saw them doing for three minutes or as long as you can keep it up! Remember, avoid repeating a movement twice in a row!

3. Now observe your feelings and perceptions. Look around slowly. What do you see that you did not see before? What do you hear, smell, touch and taste that you didn't before the exercise?

Keep in mind that physical movements in general, especially when they vary, stimulate mental development. Physical activity is a key factor in activating and preserving your brain!

The following exercise is an example of how we can plant the seeds of self-worth and self-value into our own consciousness with images.

Exercise 44 — Imaging for a Fuller Life

1. Make a tape of the following or read it — preferably aloud to yourself daily for several months.
2. Be sure that your body is as relaxed as possible before you begin.
3. You can add music if you prefer — I do.
4. As you repeat the following, bring as many of your senses into the process as you can — see, hear, touch, smell, taste and sense the meaning of the words.

- I will be harmonious and whole.
- I am choosing to engage patterns and new ways of being that will heal me and make me whole.
- I am choosing a path that may not always be easy, but one I will find the courage and strength to pursue.
- I am bringing laughter and enthusiasm to my intentionality for healing and wholing.
- I am choosing to be in a process that extends my physical health and strength.
- I am choosing to understand rather than judge or blame in my relationships.
- I am recognizing the ways in which I protect myself from deeply knowing and loving others.
- I am recognizing the ways in which I protect myself from others knowing me.
- I am experiencing my mind clearing and sharpening.
- I am experiencing myself becoming more creative.
- I find that I am increasingly able to recall my dreams.
- I am experiencing a greater sense of energy and freedom.
- I am finding more pleasure in living.
- I am experiencing more and more of that which I value in myself and others.
- I feel increasingly beautiful, strong, clear, forgiving and loving.
- I have entered a process of growth and unfolding that will always be with me.

You may wish to add or delete words or perhaps rewrite the whole experience, substituting your particular goals for yourself. Just keep in mind that you can't lie to your brain. Your intentions have to be reasonable. You also can't tell yourself that you already are all of these things.

You are in the process of becoming, which is true. The more effort, energy and creativity you put into this experience, the more impact it will have on your life!

This experience can also be danced. For more active people the addition of movement underscores and even more deeply strikes the mind.

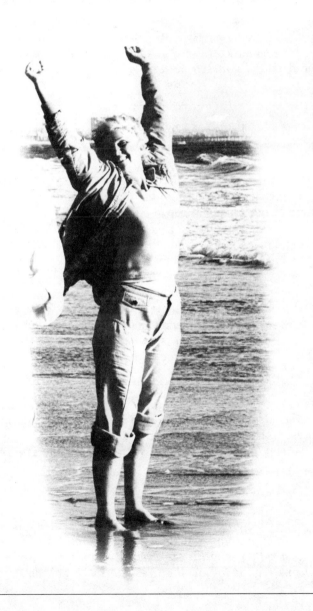

Another way to seed or impress your brain with fresh positive images has to do with selective daydreaming. We all daydream about one thing or another, so we might as well put this time to work in ways that will enhance the quality of life. Moreover, since daydreaming is a seeding and imaging process anyway, feeding our brains images that extend life will do more for us than those that reinforce hurt, anger and anxiety. Keep in mind that whatever the brain learns about life "out there" is the result of sensory input, real or, as in the case of daydreams, imagined!

Here is an exercise that will help you use your daydreams in order to understand yourself better.

Exercise 45 — Creative Daydreaming[4]

1. Make the decision to observe yourself objectively whenever you daydream. Good times to affirm your intentions to do this consistently are before you fall asleep at night and when you awaken in the morning.
2. As you observe yourself daydreaming, watch the images and messages that you're sending to your brain, and ask, "Is this what I want my brain to believe about me?"
   a. If the answer is "no." you may want to alter your daydream or change its ending.
   b. If the daydream pleases, you may wish to reinforce it by adding music and dancing to it. Remember, the more sensory material you bring to the process, the more deeply your brain absorbs the message.

Very deep relaxation can also facilitate the imaging and seeding processes. Hypnosis, self-hypnosis and autogenic training bring together these deep forms of relaxation with imaged suggestions.

The following autogenic exercise illustrates a more elaborate way of deeply relaxing yourself than earlier examples of self-relaxation did. As this is a rather lengthy exercise you may wish to put it on tape or have someone read it to you the first few times you do it.

Exercise 46 — Autogenic Exercise[5]

1. Begin by asking yourself what suggestion or image you would like to deeply implant in your brain.

    a. Select the suggestion and its wording carefully. Be sure it's something you really want for yourself.

    b. The context of the suggestion needs to be positive, otherwise you may be giving yourself a negative message. For example, if I implant the suggestion "I won't be hungry all the time," that implies that I *am* hungry *all the time!* What I want to tell my brain is that I enjoy a sense of fullness and well-being when I eat lightly.

2. Make yourself comfortable in a chair or lie down.

    a. Focus on the arm that you usually write with and feel it growing heavier and heavier. Bring three or more of your senses into this process — see, touch, smell, taste, sense its weight!

    b. Move your focus to the other arm and do the same thing. Feel it grow heavier and heavier.

    c. Now shift your attention to the leg that corresponded to the arm you began with. Feel, see, sense, etc., this leg growing heavier and heavier.

    d. Now do the same thing with the opposite leg.

3. Repeat the above only this time suggesting that your arms and legs are warm. Remember, bring in as much sense material as possible.

    a. My right arm is warm (if that's the one you began with).

    b. My left arm is warm.

    c. My right leg is warm (if that's the one you started with).

    d. My left leg is warm.

4. My arms and legs are heavy and warm. Take a moment to experience this fully.

5. Now concentrate on your breathing and repeat twice: "My breathing is full and easy. My breathing is full and easy. It breathes me."

6. Now center your attention on the area around your heart and repeat: "My heart beats evenly." Focus on the regularity of your heartbeat.

7. Shift attention to your brow and repeat: "My forehead is pleasantly cool." Repeat this twice.

8. Now imagine yourself in an idyllic setting walking alongside a body of water. Hear the birds singing, feel the warmth of the sun on your body, smell the sweet scent of the earth and air, see the beauty that surrounds you and feel yourself to be a part of all this. Reach out and make

contact with it and taste something if you wish. See a boat in the water—sturdy and very comfortable. You climb in, lie down and surrender to the gentle rock of the boat as it carries you along with the current.

9. At this deliciously relaxed point you look up in the sky and see the suggestion you intended to give yourself written in the sky. You may hear the message being spoken instead, or perhaps you both see and hear it. Let the message inform every cell in your body.

10. Once you have experienced the message you are ready to awaken. Do this slowly.

   a. Tell yourself that on the count of ten you will be awake and alert.

   b. Bring yourself up by counting to ten, feeling more awake and alert with each count.

If you wish to deepen the experience of relaxation even further at the point where your physical body is relaxed, heavy and warm, breathing full and easy, heart steady and forehead pleasantly cool, you walk down a flight of twenty stairs to the water. Since this is your fantasy, and you can do anything in it, you may wish to take an elevator or the escalator. What is important here is that you feel the sensation of moving down.

Perhaps you're finding yourself so deeply relaxed that you're falling asleep before you're able to give yourself the intended suggestion. If this is the case, the following suggestions will help:

1. Sit erect in a straight-backed chair. Don't worry if your head droops, but keep your spine straight!

2. Another way to maintain alertness is to make a "zzz" sound.

   a. Put your teeth together and make a "zzz" sound until they rattle.

   b. This sound sends blood to the brain and keeps you awake.

3. Toning or chanting briefly before you begin the deep relaxation can also be helpful in this regard.[6] Make some sighing or groaning sounds. Follow those with spontaneous tones or sounds that grow naturally in volume or turn into surging or chanting. Do this for a few minutes until you run out of steam.

If you find yourself falling asleep time and again as you do these exercises, you may wish to ask yourself the following question: "Am I exhausted or depressed? Do I feel hopeless, helpless and overwhelmed about something?" Take this question into meditation or work on it in your personal journal. There are always good reasons why we can or cannot do something.

If you find that you can't quiet your mind in the first place enough to relax, you may find it helpful to ask: "What do I feel anxious about?

What do I need to do or make happen that I'm not paying attention to?"
Dialoguing with parts that can't pay attention can also be very helpful.
(Refer to dialogue section.)

Time distortion

One of the options that you have available in the deeply relaxed state
is to distort time as your brain normally perceives it. The brain has the
capacity to function much more rapidly than we are accustomed to. An
example of this is the stories people report of seeing their whole lives flash
before their eyes in a few seconds when caught in some perilous situation.

You can suggest that a small amount of time is equivalent to a larger
amount with as much taking place in a few minutes mentally as would in
several hours or even days.

*The following exercise will help you rest deeply in a short
amount of clock time. This is a sensational practice for people on the
go who need to rest but rarely have the time to do so.*

Exercise 47 — Distorting Clock Time[4]

1. Suggest to yourself that your arms, legs and eventually whole body
is growing heavier and warmer, that your breathing is full and easy, that
your heart beats steadily, and your forehead is pleasantly cool. Follow
the format suggested in the autogenic exercise. (Refer to Exercise 46.)

2. Now visualize yourself moving slowly, consciously down a flight
of stairs, escalator, elevator, etc. Involve yourself fully in the moving down
process, seeing, hearing, touching, smelling, tasting and sensing the
experience.

3. The stairs, etc., lead to a place of beauty and safety for you. Sense
fully the comfort and pleasure of your surroundings.

4. Now tell yourself that during the next ten minutes of clock time
you will rest so deeply that it will be equivalent to an hour or two of the
deepest and most refreshing sleep. In ten minutes you will awaken fully
refreshed and revitalized. In order to insure that I am going to take ten
mintues of clock time I look at my watch and note what time it will be in
ten minutes.

Improving memory

When it comes to memory, one thing to keep in mind is that feeling deepens it and makes recall easier. That which you want to remember you'll do well to attach to some kind of emotional investment. Another way of putting this is to say that involvement that is emotional as well as intellectual is deeper and longer-lasting. Recalling events from the past is an excellent way to sharpen and extend memory in the present.

Following are two exercises that enhance memory through the recall processes.

Exercise 48 — Recalling a Day in Your Childhood[4]

1. Take a few deep breaths and relax yourself.
2. Let your mind move backward in time to the earliest age you can recall with some clarity.
3. Now follow yourself through the day at that age: See and feel yourself waking up, getting out of bed, dressing, eating, going off to school or playing. Are you doing these things alone? Who is there with you? How are you involved with the people around you?

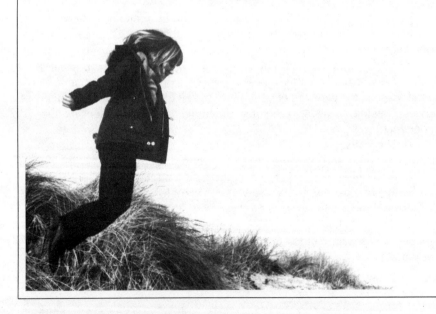

Exercise 49 — Strobe-like Recall

1. Pick a subject — any subject. Clothes, pets, cars, houses I've lived in, friends I've had, etc.
2. Now in strobe-like fashion, image scenes from your childhood past involving the subject you've chosen. Don't allow more than three seconds to go by before you change pictures. Keep this up for two or three minutes.

Do this exercise regularly once a week, while you're standing in line, shaving, setting your hair, etc.

Consciously connecting with what has been labeled unconscious[7]

When people conceptualize about the functions of the left hemisphere, words like active, verbal, logical, sequential and rational suggest themselves. When conceptualizing about the functions of the right hemisphere, words like intuitive, abstract, fantasy, unconscious and nonverbal are suggestive. Put in the simplest of contexts, the left hemisphere is the seat of rational, sequential thinking and the right, the seat of irrational, inspirational thinking. Both functions are absolutely necessary for well-being. In a technological society, the capacity to think rationally grounds us and permits us to absorb, sort through and respond appropriately to the pressures and challenges imposed by our complex lives. If the quality of life, however, is to encompass more than survival, it must include experiences that are also creative and inspirational. A full life includes the capacity to be lifted out of contexts that are practical and predictable to ones that inspire and inform us of new possibility.

In describing the two hemispheres I have of necessity used a linear verbal form and described first one half and then the other as if a choice existed between functioning one way or the other. This is not necessarily true, for the possibility exists of bringing together both kinds of thinking. In such situations we verbalize and conceptualize that which is nonverbal, unconscious and intuitive. In this society survival dictates development of left brain functioning so all of us are aligned to some degree with this kind of thinking. Those individuals who perceive themselves as artistic, intuitive and creative align themselves with right brain functions as well, although not necessarily conscious of the fact that in order to produce a work of art or affect others with intuitional insight both parts of the brain are engaged and various left and right brain processes are taking place simultaneously. Insight may occur in the right hemisphere, but it can't be expressed without the left brain functions. One is the thread off which the other spins. The rest of this section will explore rational connection to right hemisphere process-dreaming, creative expression and fantasy, but first you need to acquaint yourself with an experience of your brain that will give you the opportunity to consciously do more than one thing at a time.

The following experiences will teach you to recognize that you can and do use your brain to focus on more than one thing at a time. They will also stretch and extend your awareness significantly if you do them with some regularity.

The following exercise from the work of Robert Masters and Jean Houston demonstrates the use of both brain hemispheres simultaneously.

Exercise 50 — Left Brain/Right Brain Exercise

1. Seat yourself comfortably in a quiet setting. Take a few deep breaths and relax yourself. (Refer to Exercise 21 on deep breathing.)
2. Visualize a color, red, for example, filling the left side of your head; now visualize another color, blue, for example, filling the right side. Now be aware of both colors at the same time.
3. Hear a sound, that of the sea, for example, filling the left side of your head. Now hear a completely different sound, that of a baby crying, for example, filling the right side. Next be aware of both sounds at the same time.
4. Imagine touching something, a piece of sandpaper, for example. Think about how sandpaper feels on the left side of your brain. Now imagine touching something else on the right side, velvet, for example. Now be aware of both textures at the same time.
5. Smell a smell, coffee, for example, with the left side of your brain. Now smell another smell, vinegar, for example, with the right side of your brain. Now be aware of both smells at the same time.
6. Taste something, a fresh sweet peach, for example, and let this taste fill the left side of your head. Now taste something else, spaghetti, for example, and let this taste fill the right side of your head. Now be aware of both tastes at the same time.

7. Imagine a little red car on the left side of your brain, running round and round your brain. First it goes round and round horizontally, and then round and round vertically—then round and round every which way very fast. Now imagine a little blue car on the right side of your head doing the same thing, going round and round horizontally, vertically and every which way. Now imagine both cars meeting at the back of your throat and you swallow them!!

Here is another exercise that brings together the differing perspectives of the left and right brain in teaching or learning situations.

Exercise 51—Note-taking Using Both Halves of Your Brain

1. The next time you take notes for one reason or another, make sure that you have at least two markedly different colored pens to write with. Some people prefer to use many varying colored pens, but two is the minimum.

2. As you experience the material being presented, let yourself be aware that it is affecting you at several levels:

    a. The words convey one message. Write these down with one of the colored pens.

    b. Emotions, fantasies, creative ideas are sparked. Write these down, even those that seem very fragmentary, with the other pen.

3. Later take a look at what you have written and appreciate the complexity of your brain!

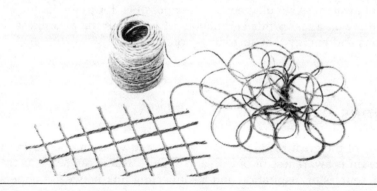

The following experience demonstrates the use of both brain hemispheres simultaneously.

Exercise 52 — Meditating on Two Objects[8]

1. Select two differing objects to hold in the palms of your hands, such as a rock and a flower, a feather and a crystal, etc.

2. Seat yourself comfortably in a quiet environment and concentrate first on the object in the hand you write with. Bring all of your senses into play during the process. Feel it, see it with your eyes closed, smell it, taste it and hear it.

3. Once you feel very familiar with, really connected to, this object, switch your attention to your other hand and the object it contains. Again direct your sensory awareness to this object.

4. Now focus very rapidly back and forth between the two until the experience of the two melts into one experience of both. Hold this awareness for a few seconds and enjoy it.

One of the things these experiences do is to extend awareness of the impartial observer in you. It is possible to dramatically alter or shift consciousness over a period of time through this kind of extension process. People try to effect awareness changes very rapidly with the use of drugs. The processes suggested here are, of course, slower. They are, however, no less effective, and have none of the dangerous side effects that drugs do.[22]

As you begin to experience the potential and flexibility of your brain, you can set the intention to use more and more of it all the time. Just as several objects can be held in your two hands and experienced simultaneously, so your brain is perfectly capable of focusing on several levels of awareness simultaneously. It is possible, for example, to concentrate on a task while simultaneously maintaining awareness of the emotions and energy that surrounds you.

Dreams

One of the great roads to the creativity and wisdom housed in the right brain is awareness of our dreams.[10] Our dreams can serve as teachers, guides, sources of inspiration and a connecting link between the personal and the universal within us. In order to learn from dreams, first you have to be able to recall them. Begin by accepting the fact that you do dream. There is absolutely no doubt that everyone normally dreams three or four times each evening. When circumstances or certain kinds of drugs interrupt this pattern, people become irritable and find it increasingly difficult to concentrate. Dreams provide a very necessary function for well-being.

Try the following exercise if you are one of those people who swears that you've never dreamed or dream only rarely.

Exercise 53 — Giving Yourself the Suggestion that You Will Remember Your Dreams

1. Use the autogenic exercise to relax yourself deeply. Suggest that you will dream tonight and remember your dreams and write them down. (Refer to Exercise 46.)
   a. See yourself dreaming, awakening and immediately writing the dream down.
   b. Make this imaging as real as possible by involving three or more of your senses. See, hear, touch, taste and smell the scene as you sleep, dream, awaken and write the dreams down immediately.
2. Before you go to bed, place paper and pen very close by so that you will hardly have to move in order to write.
   a. A tape recorder is equally effective.
   b. Be sure to include the feeling tone of the dream — do you awaken happy, sad, scared to death, etc.?
3. Don't let yourself believe that you will be able to recall your dreams without recording them immediately. You can remember a dream in great detail upon awakening and completely forget it within the next five minutes.

An alternative method of dream recall, although not necessarily as effective, is simply to say to yourself several times during the day and before bed, "I will remember my dreams this evening and record them immediately upon awakening." Again, have your recording materials close at hand while you sleep.

It is important to keep in mind as you attempt to recall dreams that you need only to remember a fragment in order to have something of value to explore. The smallest part of a dream can open doors to other parts or serve in itself as a helpful teacher and guide. Of particular importance is the feeling tone of the dream fragment, so be sure to record it.

The following exercise engages your creativity by suggesting ways to recall dreams that are particularly appropriate for you.

Exercise 54 — Meeting the Dream Master[4]

1. Deeply relax your body, using suggestions in the autogenic exercise. (Refer to Exercise 46.)

2. As you feel yourself physically becoming fully relaxed, begin a journey that takes you down a flight of twenty stairs. Count out each one as you descend into a meadow alive with the sight, sound, smell, taste and feel of spring.

3. Notice that in a clearing ahead stands a beautiful tree under which someone is seated. The seated figure is the dream master — the personification of that part of you which knows how to recall dreams. Move forward until you're close enough to see the figure clearly and make friendly contact.

4. Say that you wish help in recalling dreams, and ask for suggestions that will help you. Continue in dialogue fashion until you have secured the desired information.

5. Thank the dream master, and say that you may return again at another time for more suggestions or help with dream interpretation.

Should you have difficulty in either maintaining contact with a figure or eliciting information, keep in mind that *you are in charge.* This is a waking daydream which your brain is creating. What you believe determines what you will get. If you are insistent on making contact and getting answers, you will! Dream recall, like any other exercise or discipline, becomes easier with practice. Stay with your intention to remember dreams and keep in mind that the smallest fragment can be a jewel in terms of self-understanding.

Once you know that you do indeed dream and can recall parts if not all of your dreams, you will want to be able to understand their meaning. Understanding begins with the awareness that almost any dream can be seen from a variety of perspectives, each valid and accurate. A dream can mirror events of the day, describe disowned parts of your personality (refer to voice dialogue section in the chapter on "Extending Emotional

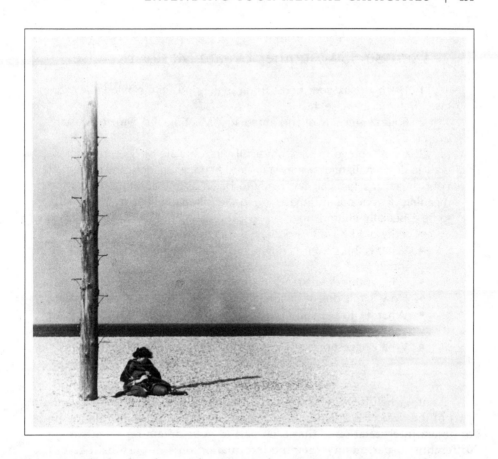

Awareness"), heal and provide a source for creative inspiration and empowerment. Dreams express a variety of messages because they come from the part of our mental process that views multidimensionally. From this it follows that there are many ways to interpret dreams. The simplest of these is simply to make an intuitive guess about the meaning of a dream based on feeling tone, your recall of the dream and the events taking place in your life. For people who feel connected to their intuition, this method works well. After all, intuitional thinking is not dissimilar from the dream process itself—both are irrational.

Unfortunately, many people do not find it particularly easy to tap into their intuitional sensing initially. One by-product, incidentally, of continuing to interpret your dreams is that this intuitional sensing grows as a result of this process. One way to interpret the material that you've collected from your dreams is to return to the dream master exercise for understanding.

The following is an adaptation of the dream master experience (refer to Exercise 54) for purposes of dream interpretation.

Exercise 55 — Another Dream Master Exercise

1. Deeply relax your body, using suggestions in the autogenic exercise. (Refer to Exercise 46.)
2. Follow steps two and three in "Meeting the Dream Master" exercise.
3. Once you've moved physically into a state of deep relaxation, walked down a flight of twenty stairs into a spring meadow and contacted your dream master, you are ready to begin asking questions about the meaning of your dream. I have found the following lines of questioning to be especially illuminating:

- Why did I have this particular dream?
- What is this dream saying to me about my life and how I'm leading it?
- What is this dream teaching me about myself and possibly others?
- How is this dream healing me?
- What is this dream showing me that I have not recognized consciously?
- What suggestions is this dream making to me?

Another helpful way to interpret dreams is to engage each character or part of the dream in a dialoging process. The assumption in this method of dream interpretation is that each part of your dream represents a different sub-personality. (See the information on sub-personalities in the chapter on "Extending Emotional Awareness.") This part can be symbolized by a person, an animal or an object such as a car or house in the dream. One by one, each is addressed in order to understand the meaning of the dream. The dialogue can take place in a deeply relaxed state, in meditation, within a personal journal or with the aid of a facilitator.

The following exercise is an example of dialogue process in meditation with dream parts.

Exercise 56 — Meditative Dialogue with Dream Parts

1. Take a few deep breaths and relax your body.
2. Go over the dream in your mind's eye as thoroughly as you can.

3. Choose a character, an object or one aspect of the dream to address first. Bring this person or thing into focus as clearly as possible and ask the following kinds of questions:

- Who are you? What are you doing in my dream?
- What part of me do you represent?
- What do you want me to know or do?
- How do you feel about other parts of this dream?
- What do you have to tell me or teach me?

If answers are unspecific or unclear, continue the dialoguing process until you are satisfied that the questions you asked have been answered to your satisfaction.

4. When you feel complete with one part, move on to another.

Remember that the dialoguing process can work equally well writing in a journal, with a facilitator or as a part of an autogenic exercise. I suggest that you experiment with several of these forms in order to find the one or ones most productive for you.

There is one more important way that dreams can be used to link consciousness with that which has been called "unconscious." This involves a process of daydreaming in order to continue or end a dream that is incomplete. By incomplete I mean a dream that leaves you up in the air. Sometimes, as in a nightmare, "up in the air" can have a very literal meaning. Most people, for example, have had falling dreams at one time or another. All nightmares have a great deal to teach us about that which we fear.

The following is an example of how a nightmare can be concluded in order to give you insight about its meaning.

Exercise 57 — Concluding a Nightmare

1. As soon as you awaken, record the dream though your wish may be to forget it.

2. Relax yourself and pick up the dream at the point where it ended. Reenter it as working fantasy.

a. This is best done with your eyes closed, lying down or in meditation.

b. If the dream has been particularly frightening, you may want someone close by listening as you work with the dream.

3. If the dream was about falling, for example, fall to the point where you hit bottom and see what you find. If the dream ends as you're about to open the coffin, open it and look inside!

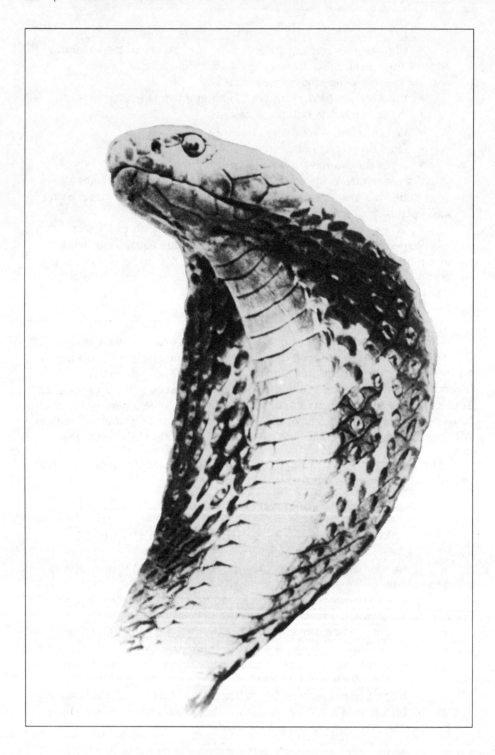

People discover their source of fear by exploring nightmares.
One nightmare understood is probably worth a year of conventional therapy!
The same process applies to dreams that may not be nightmares but feel unfinished and incomplete. Return to the dream and complete it as a fantasy. The following dream changed the dreamer's life to the extent that after she concluded the dream she experienced herself as more forceful in an ongoing way.

> The woman dreamed that there were two enormous, but perfectly harmless snakes contained within a glass room. They meant her no harm, but their size, and the fact that they were snakes, repulsed her. She awoke feeling very disgruntled before she could build up the courage to do what she knew she must, which was to enter the room with the snakes. As the woman lay in bed she determined to enter the scene in a waking fantasy. That too was surprisingly difficult. The process halted several times even though she was fully conscious. Finally she entered the room and first touched, then embraced the huge creatures. At that point the woman understood clearly that the dream was calling her attention to her need to embrace the considerable strength within her, a strength that she had previously felt was appropriate only for a man. By completing the dream as a fantasy she had in some way integrated this aspect of her personality and felt comfortable perceiving herself as both strong and feminine.

Extending creativity and the capacity to playfully explore[12]

Creativity has as much to do with playful exploration as it does profundity. All people have the capacity to be creative — to play and explore rather than imitate — though not all will bring to it the inspiration and skill that produces great art. Each time we let go judgment, expectation and control while exploring new possibilities, we become creative. This letting go is similar to the disinhibiting processes discussed near the beginning of this chapter in "Disinhibiting the brain." When old mental patterns are interrupted and brought into alignment with playful exploration, creativity is sparked. People who conceive of themselves as deficient creatively can draw, write, sing, dance and invent by engaging in processes that disrupt the usual thinking patterns. The following exercises disinhibit traditional thinking patterns and use active imagination to see the creative process. Before you begin, ask yourself, "What focus of creativity would I like to contact and develop for myself?" It could be creative writing, dance, the visual arts, music, etc. Set aside preconceptions you may have about ability with regard to this choice. Choose that which feels like it would be the most fun to do.

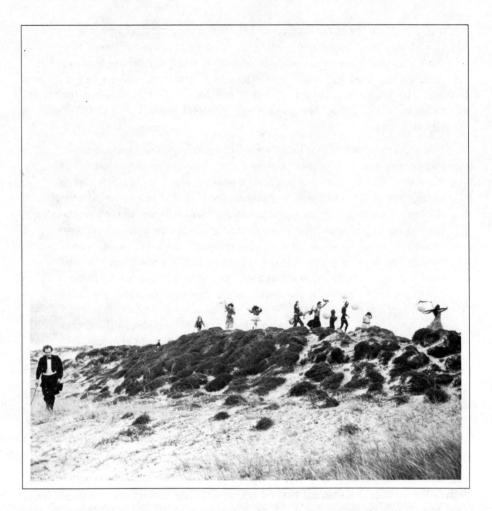

The following exercise will begin to engage your creative potential.

Exercise 58 — Creative Guide Meditation[4]

1. Move randomly and rapidly for three minutes like a three-year-old. (Refer to Exercise 43.)

2. Lie down and deeply relax following the suggestions outlined in Exercise 46 that have you experiencing your body heavy and warm, breathing evenly, heartbeat steady and forehead pleasantly cool. At this point you may wish to deepen further by descending a flight of twenty steps.

3. Tell yourself that you are now about to visit the realm of creativity and create an appropriate setting, such as a cave deep in the earth, a meadow, a forest or the seashore.

4. As you enter the realm of creativity, you meet the master teacher in the subject of your choice. Fully experience your teacher's presence. This teacher can be a real or imaginary expert on the subject you're wishing to learn about, or it can be a famous creative person from the past.

5. Tell yourself that you now have five minutes clock time which is equal to hours of imaged time in which to learn from your teacher. You may wish to enter into a dialogue or simply sit back and listen to your teacher lecture.

6. When five minutes have passed, jump up and, with the enthusiasm of a three-year-old, begin to do what your master teacher suggested.

Remember to hold a childlike, playful focus as you enter into the creative process. The point is not to produce or impress but rather to explore joyously!

Here is another exercise that is especially helpful in situations where creative blocks are experienced.

Exercise 59 — Releasing Creative Blocks

1. Begin by speaking aloud for several minutes in "make-believe language." (Refer to Exercise 38.)

2. Select a piece of music that you find particularly lively and engrossing. Lie down or dance to the music. Take the music to the stuck place and let it describe the creative process. Let it paint the picture, write the poem or invent the better mousetrap.

3. Now jump up and, holding the image of the sounds creating pictures or words, proceed with the creative process as if you and the music had become one.

The following exercise is an excellent one for slow or resistant starters because it engages your brain at a point where your body and emotional excitement may still be slumbering.

Exercise 60 — Seeding Creative Intention[4]

1. Before you fall asleep at night give yourself the suggestion that you will awaken primed for whatever creative process is your intention. Experience yourself, through active imagination, delightfully and fully involved in the process. See, hear, touch, smell and taste the experience.

2. As you awaken, experience yourself, while still in bed, fully engaged in writing, painting, inventing new formulas, etc.

3. Jump out of bed and go to it!

Keep in mind that creativity is a process, a way of being explorative — not an end product. This process is sparked and extended by playfulness, because fun and play interrupt and disinhibit patterns of judgment, expectation and control.

Part of the joyousness of this process has to do with the discovery and validation of unconscious knowing within us. We discover things about ourselves that we never dreamed of — awareness, sensitivities, feelings and thoughts that go well beyond our preconceptions about ourselves. More and more of who we are and what we have to offer others becomes knowable, and within a context of acceptance this is always wonderful!

Notes to Chapter V

[1]All of the material in this chapter was first introduced to me by Dr. Jean Houston; see R. Masters and J. Houston, *Mind Games.* The theoretical basis for the material presented in this chapter is based on the ongoing research project in Pomona, New York, that she and her husband Robert Masters support and direct. This work is substantiated by what is being called the "New Physics" — see *Brain/Mind Bulletin;* M. Ferguson, *The Brain Revolution;* B. Toben and J. Sarfatti, *Space-Time and Beyond,* for example. Therefore, I have not included footnotes for specific facts.

[2]See W. B. Joy, *Joy's Way.* This concept has been developed by Stanford researcher Dr. Karl Pribram. For an unusually clear presentation of the ideas involved, see the sixth chapter of G. Leonard, *The Silent Pulse.*

[3]Experience teaching many women's groups, as well as experience as a psychotherapist, substantiates the conclusion that this was a common experience.

[4]This exercise is a simplification and distillation of one originally taught me by Dr. Jean Houston.

[5]See H. Lindemann, *Relieve Tension the Autogenic Way;* B. Geba, *Breathe Away Your Tension;* see also R. Assagioli, *The Act of Will;* B. Samples, *The Metaphoric Mind, a Celebration of Creative Consciousness.*

[6]See L. Keys, *Toning.*

[7]See M. Ferguson, *The Brain Revolution;* J. C. Pearce, *The Crack in the Cosmic Egg;* R. Masters and J. Houston, *Mind Games;* N. Calder, *The Mind of Man;* A. Smith, *Powers of Mind.*

[8]This is an adaptation of an exercise that comes out of the Research Clinic at the Center for the Healing Arts.

[9]See B. Payne, *Getting There Without Drugs.*

[10]See M. Fay, *The Dream Guide;* J. Katz, *Dreams Are Your Truest Friends;* C. G. Jung, *Memories, Dreams, Reflections;* F. Perls, *Gestalt Therapy Verbatim.*

[11]See R. K. Dentan, *The Semai: A Nonviolent People of Malaya.*

[12]My husband, Robert Segal, and I gave a series of workshops on creativity privately and for the Association for Humanistic Psychology. I continue to be a practicing artist and worked professionally for ten years as a potter before going into the field of psychology.

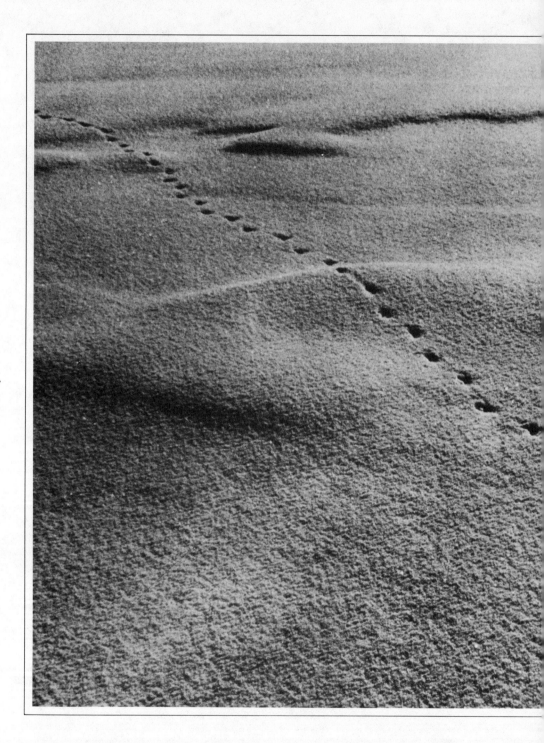

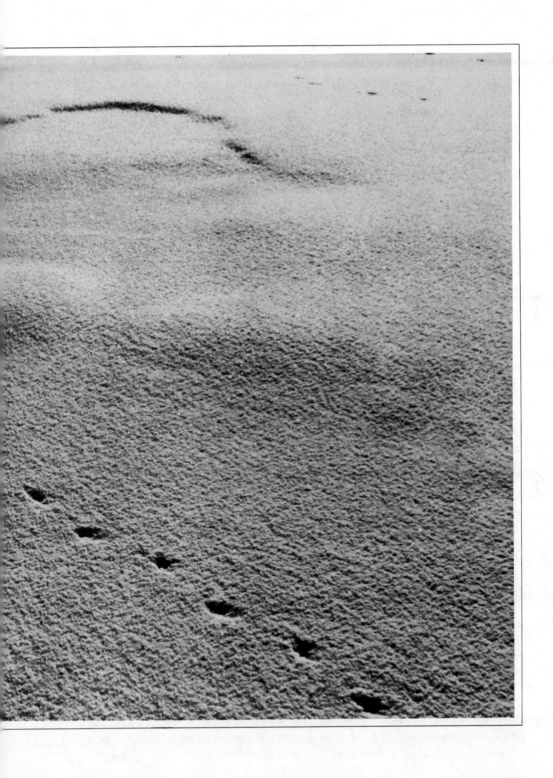

6

Extending Spiritual Awareness

Idefine spirituality as the awareness of oneself in harmony with the universe. This experience of being at one with someone or something outside of ourselves is joyous, uplifting and often emotionally touching. Ecstasy is the word that brings these feelings together for me.[1] Almost everyone, including those who are scientifically oriented, has at one time or another been moved to tears or near tears by a profoundly beautiful sunset, a piece of music, a dramatic scene or an overwhelming feeling of love for another person. At these moments, the loneliness and isolation of self-contained awareness dissolves and for a time, perhaps only a second, the impact of truly being connected to something or someone other than ourselves is experienced. And at exactly the same moment, paradoxically, we also become more deeply connected to ourselves.

Perception opens like the pages of a book and that which a moment earlier was unknown, unseen and unclear becomes knowable. In this context, our inner worlds and our outer worlds become indistinguishable from one another and all take on a profound naturalness and appropriateness. The extension of awareness may or may not be experienced as a dramatic personal event. The point is that there is no one way to respond to this extension of perception that is spiritual awareness. All that one can be sure of is that spiritual awareness, when integrated into daily living, makes even the best of lives profoundly more meaningful.

Ecstasy is not the exclusive domain of the mystic, it is a state of awareness slumbering in each of us, and it can be pursued realistically in the midst of a full, busy and materially productive life. It doesn't necessitate a large commitment or change in lifestyle. What is required is nothing more or less than the capacity to suspend disbelief in order to explore new possibilities. It is not necessary to suspend disbelief permanently. *Letting go the judgments and limitations attached to rational beliefs for only a brief time permits us to experience new learning that can lead to ecstatic well-being.*

And I may add that these states are not dependent on the use of drugs.[2] As we all know, drug use can have side effects. Moreover, the ecstatic experiences that come to one in a drug-free state are easier to hold on to. They don't disappear when the effects of the drug wear off. As such these states of consciousness can be integrated into our lives in an ongoing way that doesn't interfere with material activities. In fact, our focus on practical pursuits is strengthened by the pursuit of that which brings harmony and balance into our lives. It's true that by disinhibiting doubts, drug experiences can open one to new potentials. However, if we are willing to suspend judgment and doubts long enough to be open to a new experience, then we need not rely on drugs.

When people avoid the exploration of new possibilities, they usually do so in order to protect themselves. Sometimes the protections are rational, but more often the protections are based on unwarranted fear: fear of appearing foolish, fear of failing, fear of not measuring up or being inadequate, fear of losing something we value, etc. Sometimes the fear has to do with the loss of the ecstatic experience itself.

The following exercise can help you explore some of the reasons you may have for avoiding spiritual investigation.

Exercise 61 — Blocks to Spiritual Exploration

1. Relax yourself. (Refer to Exercise 21 or other suggestions for de-stressing.)
2. Now imagine yourself in a state of ecstasy using either an ecstatic memory from your past or an intensely joyous piece of music to help you return to that experience.
   a. Beethoven's "Ode to Joy" from the Ninth Symphony or the "Gloria" from Handel's *Messiah* are examples of stirring, ecstasy-evoking music.
   b. If you are having a hard time recalling moments of intense joy, let your memory move back to those times when as a young child you felt free, times when fearlessly you abandoned yourself to experiences, shouting, singing or swinging in the wind.
3. See yourself as you are now moving through life in this ecstatic state. Do this for a few minutes.

4. Now answer the following questions as you continue to visualize:
   a. What happens to me?
   b. What dangers are involved in being this way?
   c. Who could get hurt? How?
   d. Am I afraid of failing?
   e. Do I like it? Why? Why not?
5. To what extent are the apprehensions, if I have any, realistic?

The question that comes up again and again as we pursue our potential for well-being is "what do we really want?" When what we want most is to experience this potential, then we will begin a process that sets aside our fear-based protections in order to do it.

Spiritual meditation

Meditation is no more exotic than play. Like play, meditation is a creative process that requires no props or extended time commitment and it may be accompanied by vigorous movement. Moreover, it's fun in that "doing it" results in our feeling better and better. Real people become spiritual meditators, busy materially focused people who punch time clocks, or care for young children, or go to school.

The meditations discussed in this book, up to now, have been described in reference to their beneficial effects on the physical body—benefits that occur from relaxing and de-stressing. In addition to increased physical well-being, meditation can also open and extend spiritual awareness.[3] New perspectives are encountered when we focus on extending our usual state of consciousness. When we do this, meditation becomes a vehicle for experiencing wisdom and creativity. Why this happens, how this happens, is still speculation, but it appears to have something to do with the alpha state that takes place when we have relaxed and released to the point where our usual thinking patterns have been quieted. The alpha state represents a shift in brain wave pattern and can be felt experientially as a very deep relaxing of the physical body, which leads not to sleepiness but to an increase in energy or vitality. More profound forms of meditation can be experienced as a dissolving of the self-contained and self-conscious awareness we experience most of the time. They can also be associated with a melting and joyous intensity not unlike orgasm. It's no wonder that in many parts of the world where day-to-day living is difficult and unpleasant, spiritual meditation is the preferred way of being.

Meditation can become simply another form of escape and as such will not support a process of holistic integration. There is a difference

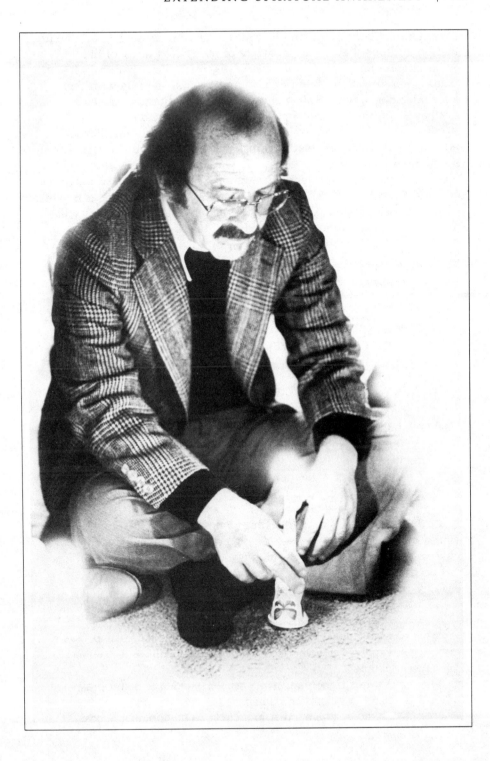

between a meditation that simply removes us from an uncomfortable life situation and one that makes us aware of the shared unity of life.

Meditation for purposes of escaping is much like a pain pill. It can deaden other aspects of living and, in any event, leaves us with the problem we began with. Spiritually extending meditation ignites an awareness that is continuous and sustained throughout the day.

When the feelings of love and joy that can be felt in meditation are sustained, and affect our relationships with other people and with life in general, then meditation can become a way of life that acts as a template or pattern for joyous experience throughout the day. Again, so much has to do with intention. When our intention is to use meditation as a vehicle to enhance the overall quality of life for ourselves and others, we will explore a process that increasingly brings this about.

The following suggestions may help to extend and involve you more intensely in spiritual meditation.

Exercise 62—Deepening Processes that Can Lead to Spiritual Meditation

1. Clear your mind and deeply relax. (Refer to the section on "Meditation" in the chapter on "Extending Physical Awareness.")
2. Very, very subtle physical movements facilitate moving into an alpha state.
   a. As you meditate, move your head, almost imperceptibly, from side to side.
   b. As you meditate, barely move a toe or finger.
3. Experiment with the length of time you meditate. Some people need much more time in order to let go completely. There may be days or periods of time when meditation is more difficult and additional time is needed to relax sufficiently.
4. Meditating with others can deepen our experience.
   a. This is especially true when we are with more experienced meditators.
   b. Meditating in groups facilitates our meditative experience. Experiment with different people and different numbers of people.
   c. Try gently holding hands as you meditate. Some prefer left hand up, right hand down.
   d. Sit facing one another in a circle, gently holding hands.

5. Sounds and music can deepen meditative concentration. (Refer to the suggestions for using music in Exercise 18.)
   a. Explore the use of various meditation tapes and records that are commercially sold.
   b. Explore the use of various kinds of music and sounds.
   c. Experiment with the effect singing and chanting or making sounds has on the meditative process for you.
   d. Let the sound come from deep within and fill you with its resonance.
   e. After you feel complete in your singing, chanting or sounding, remain quiet and receptive to whatever you may experience for a few minutes.

6. Spiritual meditation is intensified by the visualization of intense white light entering at the crown of our heads and filling our entire bodies.

7. Prayer as an adjunct to the experience of very deep relaxation can intensify meditation. Try chanting or singing the prayer aloud.

8. If you should feel uncomfortably light-headed as you complete a meditation, simply focus on the lower parts of your body. Bring awareness to your legs and feet, stamp a few times or put pressure on your toenails with your thumbs. You can also just sit quietly for a few minutes in a chair, palms down on thighs, feet apart on the floor, thinking of energy flowing from the palms of your hands and the bottoms of your feet, connecting you with the earth. These practices will direct perception and energy to the more familiar parts of your body. In time you will feel as comfortable experiencing energy in the upper parts of your body as in the lower.

In extending and expanding meditation, it is vital to focus on your process as you explore new possibilities. The process of exploration must in itself be joyous. If it is not, if it is a burden or unpleasant, then don't do it! When you have a specific goal in mind, than an intensive experience is less likely to happen. Ecstasy, like orgasm, is not something you can insist on. It occurs most frequently when involvement is with the wonder and pleasure of the process, and when it comes, it's always an amazing surprise and unlike anything you've experienced before.

Working with energy

Perceiving in terms of energy begins to soften perception of ourselves as finite and enclosed. Since matter and energy are convertible, contemporary laws of physics suggest that we, as energy, may not solely be contained within skin-bound limitations. Energy moves freely through solid matter; therefore, when we begin to perceive of ourselves as energy, we also begin to experience ourselves extending into the space around our bodies. The practical benefit of doing this in terms of well-being is that we feel lighter, healthier, more energetic and increasingly aware of our needs and the needs of others.

A consciousness of ourselves as extended beings lends support to feeling of connection and an awareness of intimate relationship with the universe. Those experiences that I categorize as "energy work" introduce us to this awareness. One of the simplest and yet most astounding demonstrations of the fact that we extend beyond our physical bodies has to do with consciously and intentionally touching the energy that extends beyond the periphery of our skins. This energetic extension is composed, at least initially, of ions, which are electrically charged particles. They are seen by increasing numbers of people and are, to some extent, photographable and therefore scientifically verifiable.

The advent of Kirlian photography has made available on film that which, in the past, only mystics could lay claim to seeing. Perhaps this accounts for the fact that today auras, the name given these energy fields, are seen by many people.

The experience of perceiving through touch the energetic fields that emanate from physical bodies is no less commonly available. Most people can learn to attune their sense of touch to the subtle awareness that permits us to experience energy emanting from the body.

The following exercises are simple examples of how to begin sensing energy fields.

Exercise 63 — Experiencing Your Own Aura [4]

1. Stand with arms open at about shoulder level and palms facing one another.
2. Close your eyes, take a few deep breaths and intend in your mind's eye to suspend disbelief, to be open to new possibilities, for a few minutes.
3. Now very, very slowly begin to bring your palms together.
4. Stop at the point where (1) your hands begin to tingle, (2) you feel heat or (3) you perceive an increase in the density of space you are moving through.

5. Open your eyes and observe the distance between your palms. This distance is filled by your aura!

Exercise 64—Experiencing Another Person's Aura

1. Ask someone to stand at a right angle to you, and not touch you. Their left or right shoulder should be approximately eighteen to twenty-four inches from your chest.

2. In the position of the preceding exercise, with arms open at shoulder level, palms facing one another, begin moving your arms together. Keep your eyes closed and move *very, very slowly.*

3. Stop when (1) you feel a tingling in your palms, fingers or hands, (2) you feel heat, or (3) you perceive an increase in spatial density.

4. Now very, very slowly, keeping your hands in contact with your partner's energy field, move up and down your partner's body without physically touching it. Some areas may feel warmer or more dense or more tingling than others.

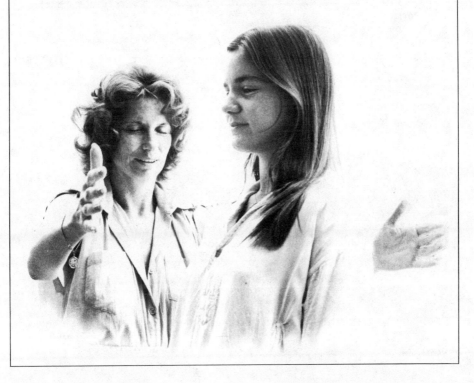

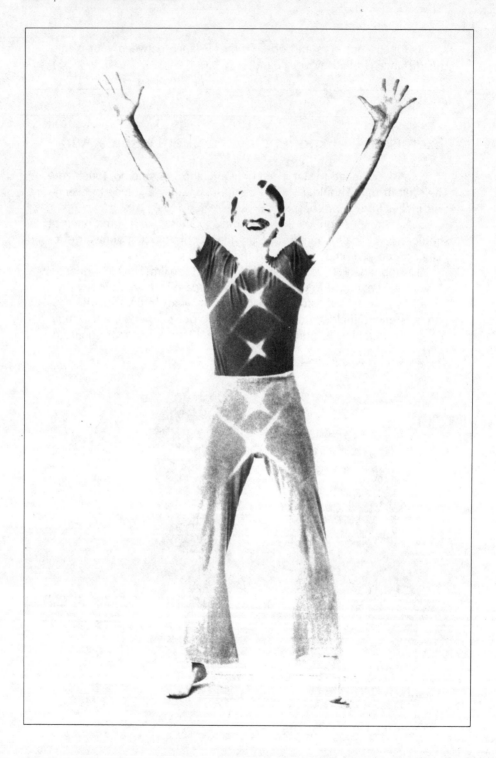

As you start to feel comfortable with the idea that energy boundaries may extend beyond initial sensory impressions, you may open to the possibility of experiencing differently the energies contained within the body, and outside the body. In the Orient a system for conceptualizing energy has existed for thousands of years that recognizes special energy clusters within the body. There is some disagreement about the number of these centers; seven are usually identified, but other schools of thought identify more. The major energy centers, called chakras, lie approximately along the spine, behind the eye sockets and at the top of the skull. Again, practical benefits of opening chakras in terms of well-being have to do with the great amounts of physical and emotional stress that can be released in this process.

The following is a meditative exercise that allows you to begin exploring with energy in new ways.

Exercise 65 — Introduction to the Chakras [5]

1. Imagine that within your body, there are seven major centers from which energy radiates or emanates beyond the skin. The seven energy centers or chakras correspond to nerve centers and glands in the physical body.

   a. The first lies at the very base of the spine between the anus and genitals.
   b. The second is located from two to three inches below the navel.
   c. The third lies in the area of the solar plexus two to three inches above the navel.
   d. The fourth lies mid-chest, at heart level.
   e. The fifth is located in the throat.
   f. The sixth lies in the head between the eyebrows.
   g. The seventh is located at the crown of the head.

2. In addition to these seven energy centers or vortices, there is also an eighth major center that lies about eighteen inches above the crown. There are also important centers of energy in the knees and feet. Simply let your imagination accept these as possibilities.

The following is an exercise that draws attention to these subtle energies. It will also help to stimulate and intensify the releasing of these energies.

Exercise 66 — Opening Your Chakras

1. Sit with your spine erect or lie down flat in a comfortable position (don't fall asleep though!).

2. Put your attention on the area about eighteen inches above your head. Imagine a sphere about the size of a tennis ball radiating clear white light. This light penetrates the top of the skull igniting the chakra in this area.

    a. If pictures or thoughts interrupt your focus first, let them pass on by.

    b. Focus on the feeling of openness and expansion for a minute or so before moving on to the next chakra.

    c. If you experience little or nothing at first, don't be discouraged. One area may be easier for you to identify and open than another at first.

3. Now move on to the area between the brows. Repeat the steps above.

4. Move on, exploring the throat chakra, the heart chakra, the chakra near the solar plexus, the abdomen chakra a few inches below your navel, and the root chakra at the body base. Take as much time as you need at each chakra.

5. If you experience an uncomfortable sense of light-headedness, sit quietly for a time directing attention to your feet, the floor or the chair you're sitting on. Stamping or dancing can also be helpful in this regard. Keep in mind that the perception of lightness can intensify focus and mental clarity.

6. Because of the complexity of this experience, a tape recorder or a friend who will read the directions would be helpful.

At this point, if you've completed the exercise, you may feel a sense of expansion. If you had taken a Kirlian photo before and after the exercise, the film would validate your awareness. You have indeed extended your energetic body and lightened your physical body.

Occasionally, the release of energy triggers the release of emotions and people want to cry or laugh. Go ahead, but keep in mind that the release of emotion, while beneficial, is not the same as the release of energy that leads to spiritual awareness. Unexpressed emotion can block the pursuit of spiritual perception. Emotional release is therefore beneficial, and often results in good feelings, but these feelings do not represent spiritual awareness.

It is important to keep in mind that all of the exercises in this book, and particularly those that have to do with energy, are intended to be practiced in a drug-free state. *There is nothing drugs do for us that we are not capable of doing for ourselves in the pursuit of spiritual ecstasy.*

Attuning to light

Perception of reality grows richer and more interesting as mental control, stress and tension are released. The capacity to experience intensely also grows so that if the focus we choose is positive, our experiences grow increasingly wonder-full. One of the most exquisite experiences that is available to us has to do with the perception of a subtle source of energetic nourishment that surrounds us. This source is perceived in the form of light, and anyone can attune themselves to it. The experience of light does not require years of training or hours of meditation. I have seen ordinary people completely unfamiliar with mind-extending processes align themselves with this source of light. What is necessary is the suspension of disbelief.

The following exercise can introduce you to the subtle awareness of light that is in relationship with you.

Exercise 67—Connecting with the Source of Light That Lies Beyond Your Physical Body

1. Begin at a point where you have already opened the seven chakras.
2. Before continuing, focus on the minor energy centers in the knees and feet.
   a. Open one knee at a time, as you did the other areas.
   b. Now turn your attention to your feet and open the energy, first in one foot and then the other.
3. Now give your focused attention to the area about eighteen inches above the crown of your head. Imagine a particularly brilliant white light at this point, which enters, fills and extends you still more.

Allow the experience of this brilliant light to affect you. Surrender to it and allow whatever comes.

    a. Set aside for a few minutes your disbelief.

    b. If you feel frightened of letting go, acknowledge the fear.

    c. Hold the sensation without analyzing or categorizing it.

This state of awareness can lead to particularly profound experiences when you introduce your inner guide at this point. Don't be surprised if your guide changes form. (In fact, your guide may lose form entirely.)

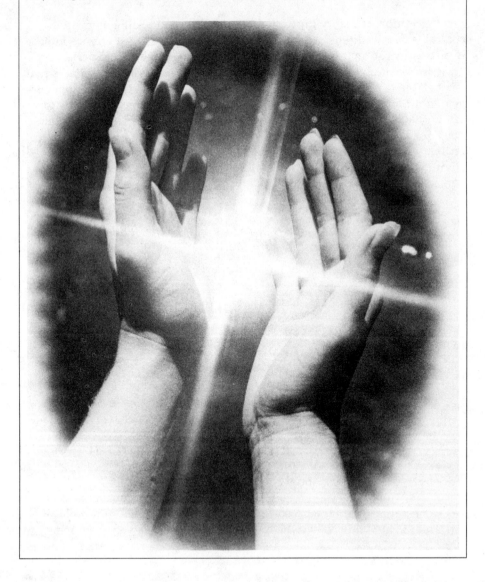

The following exercise will lead to a less controlled, more dreamlike guide meditation.

Exercise 68 — Extended Guide Meditation[4]

1. Once you have opened your energy centers and are experiencing a sense of light that lies outside of you and yet penetrates your body, ask to experience your guide. (Refer to Exercise 58.)
    a. Remember, at this time your guide may not come to you as he or she did in the past.
    b. In any event, let whatever happens be received with openness and acceptance.
2. You may wish to experience your guide passively, simply receiving whatever messages the guide brings, or you may wish to ask questions and obtain specific information from your guide concerning a problem or decision that you need to make. Dialogue with your guide can sometimes be facilitated by having someone else present.
3. If as you resume your activities you feel a bit light-headed, refocus on your legs and feet. Jump, stamp or dance around until you feel surefooted. As you concentrate on the upper parts of your body, energy is drawn to those parts. Refocusing on lower parts brings the energy back down so that you feel more grounded.

Developing the skill of subtle sensing

All of your senses are capable of being more fully developed. Heightened consciousness results from this heightening of the senses. Day-to-day awareness takes on whole new dimensions that extend well-being as we experience ourselves creative, intense and deeply connected to others and to our own individuality at one and the same time. Well-being takes on added pleasurable dimensions when we perceive more. We become smarter, more creative, more deeply feeling, more responsive and therefore more able to love and be loved. Energetic experiences that are explored with increasing frequency become increasingly concrete and available.

Opening the subtler senses
with music[7]

Music is probably one of the most available bridges for the activation of the subtler senses because we hear not only with our ears, but our entire body as well. The skin is a sensing organ containing countless receptors that respond to changing vibrations. Deaf individuals experience music as shifting vibrations. Classical music almost always includes a much greater variety of sounds, and is therefore more stimulating than musical forms that are more limited in range. This is not to say that classical music is the only music with a wide range of sound frequencies.

Volume affects the intensity of the sound vibration. The louder the music, the more acutely we experience its vibrations. Sound is thus capable of stimulating and awakening receptors in the skin that feed us the information upon which perception is based. As more information is received, more of what we call reality is experienced, and with it the possibility of extending awareness of ourselves, of our relationship to others and of the universe.

The following exercise will introduce you to the possibility of awakening subtler sensing with high intensity sound.

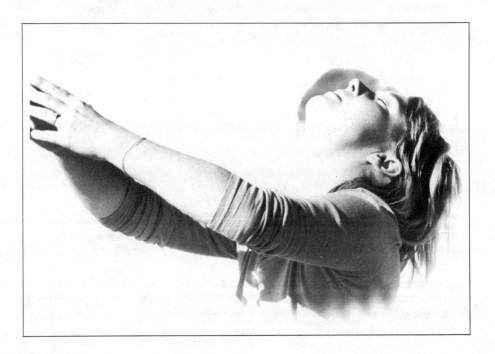

Exercise 69 — Experiencing Sound Intensity

1. Select a piece of music that contains a wide range of sounds — some very high, and others very low.
   a. The classics, because of their variety of instrumentation, usually include a wide range of sound frequencies.
   b. Some selections are generally more evocative than others. Pachelbel's "Canon in G" is especially moving.
   c. The intent is to experience each note as if you were hearing it for the first time. Therefore, very familiar music is *less* likely to make an impact, as there is a tendency to get involved with it mentally.

2. Turn up the volume as high as you can bear or dare! (Consider inviting family or roommates to share this experience with you, rather than having to worry about disturbing whatever else they might be doing.)

3. Lie on the floor, palms down and surrendering to its intensity. Let the sound enter you.

4. Allow whatever happens to be experienced with acceptance. If your response is emotional, and you feel like crying or laughing, go ahead!

5. Give yourself a few minutes to slowly get up. If you feel lightheaded, and that's inappropriate for what you need to do next, jump up and down or dance, focusing the return of energy to your feet.

6. If your body vibrates, allow it.

Extending your sense of sight

Most of the time we focus precisely on that which we are looking at, as if all that we wished to see consisted of fine print. Precision and absolute clarity is valued, and if our vision refuses to conform to this valuing we correct and recorrect with lenses until absolute clarity is insured. Sensitized and extended vision is, however, brought about by relaxing the focus of the eyes. As we soften our gaze, much more input is received. A much vaster picture is experienced, one that may leave us with the impression of seeing not only that which is directly in front of us, but to the side and behind as well.

Soft eyes or a relaxed gaze also permit us to see phenomena that are not perceived when visual focus is precise. The energy fields that surround the body are more likely to be seen when we soften our gaze, although this requires practice.

The following exercise can introduce you to the possibility of extending your visual sensitivity.

Exercise 70 — Relaxed Gazing

1. Select a setting for this exercise that is visually unexciting, such as a plain room with white or light walls and indirect lighting. Ask someone to sit or stand in front of a blank wall and position yourself across from them.
2. Relax yourself by taking a few deep breaths.
3. Focus your attention on the internal sensations in your own body, relaxing and releasing any tension you may notice.
4. Now direct your gaze to the person sitting across from you in front of the blank wall.
   a. Relax your vision.
   b. Rather than gazing directly, look out of the sides of your eyes.
   c. Allow whatever feelings may accompany this process to be experienced with acceptance.
5. Suspend disbelief and allow yourself to experience whatever you may see.

You may see nothing that you have not seen before when you do this exercise, and that's perfectly all right. In time, if you choose to continue to soften your gaze, you will begin to see more and more. It takes time to develop subtle sensing, particularly with senses that have not been exercised much in the first place.[6]

Extending your skill of subtle sensing

You can further validate your experience of the existence of subtle energy centers by perceiving them in other people as well as yourself.

The following exercise will begin to give you a sense of the energetic dimensions of others.

Exercise 71 — Exploring the Subtle Energy of Others [4]

1. Have your partner lie down, on a table if that is possible.

2. Very, very slowly move your hand over their body. Begin with the hand you normally write with, for maximum sensitivity. Your hand should be from two to six or eight inches above them.

3. When you perceive the slightest variation, stop and open your eyes as you slowly pass over the body.

    a. Where is your hand? Are you near or over one of the chakra energy centers?

    b. Do the experiment first with one hand and then the other.

    c. Try the experience palm up and palm down.

4. At first you may perceive only the faintest change, but if you continue, your sensitivity will increase. Let yourself believe in it — allow yourself to accept the possibility that what you think you're feeling is "really there."

This exercise is training your subtle sense of touch just as you would train your ear by repeated listening. You will also discover that some individuals are much easier to scan in this way than others. This, of course, has to do with the degree to which their energy centers are open.

Affirmation and positive intentionality

Profound meditations, and experiences of intense and joyous connection with other people and the universe, acquaint us with moments of ecstasy. These come, for most, infrequently, and leave quickly. The pressures and distractions of contemporary living are partially responsible for this, but it also has to do with the belief system that requires our being "on guard" most of the time. Many individuals put tremendous amounts of energy into protecting themselves from other people and from life in general. Experience has taught them that they can be hurt, and life is lived with that expectation and the protections that cover it.

The following exercise will heighten your awareness in regard to your particular belief system.

Exercise 72 — Is the Universe Friendly?

1. Make yourself comfortable sitting or lying down and take a few deep breaths.

2. Ask yourself the following questions with as much detachment as possible:

    a. Is the universe personally friendly, unfriendly or indifferent to me? If your choice was "indifferent," ask: "What is the difference between an indifferent and an unfriendly universe?"

    b. Why do I believe the universe to be friendly, unfriendly, indifferent?

    c. At what age did I first view the universe as friendly, unfriendly or indifferent?

    d. Is the choice I first made about the relative friendliness of the universe valid today?

    e. Do I want to stick with my choice?

3. If you believe the universe to be unfriendly or indifferent, ask the following question: "How do I protect myself from the hostility or coldness of this unfriendly or indifferent universe?"

4. Accept whatever conclusions you have drawn from this exercise about your belief systems. They represent an honest evaluation of your beliefs at this moment. Recall that positive change and growth usually begin best with awareness and acceptance of where you're starting from!

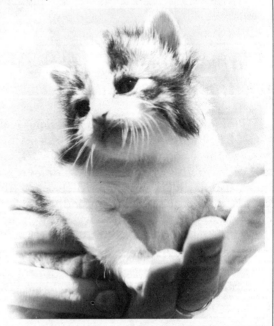

If your evaluation of the universe is negative, or somewhat negative, keep in mind that you can genuinely acknowledge and accept these views because in the past they have led to protections for good reasons. Few would want to commune with a universe that is unfriendly or even indifferent. The consequence, however, of protections is that they block energy and the experiences that lead to spiritual awareness.

Focus on affirmation and positive intention are two ways of balancing the fear and subsequent energy blocking behaviors that many are attached to. Our experience depends, to a great extent, on what we choose to focus on. I can continue to think about the frustrations of the day or I can concentrate on something that gives me pleasure such as running, my children's bright faces, the sunset, etc. Do I choose to give attention to my disappointments, worries and expectations, or do I choose to focus on processes that lead to well-being? When we intend to feel good, the balancing process that gives attention to physical, mental, emotional and spiritual aspects of life facilitates this. The choice, however, always lies in the moment. By this I mean that negative assumptions about oneself, others and life in general will present themselves in our consciousness from time to time. In these moments we have a choice to make that will lead to either an increase or a decrease in well-being. The enhancing choice we make may not necessarily produce happy feelings instantly, but it will tend to increase overall well-being.

The following exercises can help to facilitate the choice to feel well when we are feeling badly. This exercise can be done in written form, but I believe that it is most effective as a verbal statement to another person or in prayer.

Exercise 73 — List of Appreciations

1. Relax yourself. (Refer to Exercise 21 and other suggestions for de-stressing.)

2. Reflect on the people and events that bring you pleasure and joy.

3. As you list them, sense as fully as possible the pictures and feelings of pleasure you associate with these people and events.

4. Acknowledge your gratitude.

5. Consciously choose to hold this state of awareness throughout the day.

That which we believe we want, increasingly comes to us as we focus our desire for ecstatic well-being.

Unconditional love and the opening of energy at heart level

The most important experience in regard to spiritual awareness occurs as we engage in a process of exploration and opening that introduces us more and more to the deeply touching energy gathered in the chest at about heart level. Love is the word most choose to use in describing the emotional feeling that accompanies the physical impression of opening and expending at heart level. There is a quality of detachment, however, about this kind of love feeling that is unusual for most. One feels deep, "love" without necessarily having a specific focus for the feeling; and even when a "loved one" or "loved ones" are connected to the feeling, they are loved in a way that is independent of need, and far less personally possessive and demanding than before the heart opening. For this reason, love experienced in this way is referred to as unconditional. Desires to control and change others are softened and stoic tolerance in regard to others gives way to appreciation and acknowledgment in the context of feeling radiant and expansive.

The experience of unconditional love is a process. Awareness can come in an instant, but awareness is only the beginning of the journey. Feelings of warmth, clarity and expansion that accompany sensations of opening and releasing energy at heart level come and go for most, at least initially. Further, as time goes by, the beauty and intensity of the awareness grows. Transformation is never a "trip." It is rather an ongoing process greatly facilitated by joy that comes from self-acceptance and the putting aside of blame.

The following exercise can facilitate the process of opening energy at heart level.

Exercise 74 — Opening the Heart

1. Begin by tapping into your subtler senses. Try each of the following:
   a. If a site of great beauty is available to you, contemplate its magnificence as you sit or walk in it.
   b. An alternative beginning would be the experiencing of music described in Exercise 18 or Exercise 69.

c. Another alternative beginning would be to sing or dance joyously for a period of time.

2. Concentrate attention in your chest at heart level. As you feel yourself being moved by these experiences, focus on the warmth, excitement, tingling, etc., that is produced.

3. Hold this awareness even if it frightens you. Breathing deeply can relax and calm the scared feelings that sometimes come with the focusing of so much energy.

4. Allow and accept whatever happens.

The flooding of energy at heart level brings with it an intensity that many perceive as new and frightening. The tendency may therefore be to immediately intellectualize what happened, to talk and think about it in a way that analyzes, defines and limits the experience. It is indeed possible to speak without disengaging from the experience, but it takes willingness to maintain the focus at heart level even as you speak. Speech is thus far less rationally controlled.

The surfacing of denied emotions

It is not uncommon for intense emotions to surface as individuals begin to acknowledge the awareness of unconditional love and the sensation of opening.[8] Emotions, which include fear and pain as well as emotional ecstasy, are appropriate and should be received with acceptance. The blocks that limit our possibilities have to be exposed and accepted before they can be released. Integration is the result of acknowledgment and acceptance. These however, are only the beginnings of a consciousness that includes much more than emotional awareness. If you find yourself uncomfortable emotionally, explore the following possibilities in order to reestablish a balanced perspective.

1. Engage in strenuous physical exercise.

2. Use your journal to create a dialogue between the emotions you are feeling and your center or ego. (Refer to Exercise 29.)

3. Dialogue with your emotions in meditation or consult your inner guide. (Refer to Exercise 30 or Exercise 58.)

4. Use your dreams to bring you understanding. Ask for clarification and guidance in your dreams as you prepare to fall asleep. (Refer to Exercise 54.)

Service — the expression of unconditional love[9]

When we love unconditionally, it becomes impossible to ignore the people and conditions that surround us everywhere in the world. Moreover, the development of our subtler senses makes it very clear that the dividing line between "them" and "us" is very fine indeed. We experience directly the effect of other people's thoughts, feelings and energy. We are touched and moved by all that surrounds us, and there is no doubt about the fact that this sharing is intimate, personal and has a profound effect on our well-being. Moreover, the unconditional love we extend to others fills us with well-being, and a sense of purpose and possibility where none may have existed before. In this respect giving to others is a mutually healing and life-enhancing process. The aspect of unconditional love that prompts an extension of the self for the benefit of others I call service. Service, in this sense, is never a chore or a giving up of one's own best interest. It is rather an experience of "giving to get" from the process itself. This is not unlike the work involved in caring for your own body. Discipline, time and energy are required in order to keep physically fit, but the process becomes its own reward because it is purposeful and pleasurable. Service is not something you engage in for honor or praise; it is something you do because it feels good to you as you are doing it.

The key to the difference between sacrifice and service lies in the experience of the process. Sacrifice does not feel good, service does. I recently had the experience of spending a significant amount of time in a very busy schedule with a family member who was slowly dying. I count the experience as a privilege and one of the high points in my life. I learned more that is worthwhile about life than I have in years in the process of simply being with this man.

All of us have the capacity to extend the quality of life for others as well as ourselves. Furthermore, just as well-being requires active participation on our part in regard to self-care and self-understanding, so too, well-being requires active participation aimed at enhancing the quality of life for other people and the planet. In a very concrete way all that is "out there" touches, affects and contributes to the way we perceive life. When awareness is extended to include the experiences discussed in this section it becomes clear that the little skin-bound "self" is only part of the picture. Each individual is also participating in a greater body. The more perfectly that greater body functions, the more perfectly the skin-bound "self" functions. There are countless ways to serve others and ourselves. We can serve as healers and as creators of objects and experiences that enhance the quality of life. We can serve socially and politically to extend consciousness and the well-being of others. We can wash dishes or paint a "Mona Lisa." In terms of the value of one service over another, as we are speaking of it here, it really does not matter. What is important is the process. When the experience of serving feels good to us as well as those we serve, then we are on the right track.

In the following exercise, you can extend your awareness of the significance of process in service.

Exercise 75 — Discerning the Difference between Duty and Service

1. The next time you have a "duty" to perform — a call or visit to be made, a ride to be given, etc. — focus on the upcoming event.
2. Relax yourself and open your heart chakra. (Refer to Exercise 74.)
3. In the context of this extended state of consciousness, determine a process in the exercise of this "duty" that could afford you pleasure.
4. Now take a chance and experiment by following through with what came to you.

Most service is, of course, not undertaken as a duty once awareness of the pleasurable possibility that can lie in process is experienced. Service also affords the opportunity to do something concrete with the energy that can pour in as the heart opens. Service thus grounds the experience of unconditional love and gives it a permanent place in day-to-day life. It provides an ongoing channel for expanding energy in the midst of active worldly pursuits.

Healing as a form of service

One of the simplest and most touching forms of service is connected to healing. We are each of us healers in the sense that we can, if we choose, positively affect others with loving, unconditional energy. Anyone who has ever calmed and relaxed a hurt or frightened child knows the power of an accepting embrace. We naturally come to the aid of distressed infants and children, not only our own, but those of others — yet we hesitate when it comes to reaching out to other adults regardless of the fact that adult distresses can be as intense as any child's. The following experience will give you an idea of the healing and calming effect your unconditional energy can have on another person. Before you begin, acknowledge that the loving and healing energy you will be directing not only belongs to you, but is shared universally.

You may wish to conceive of this energy as a light source coming from God, or benevolent forces in the universe, or a higher frequency energy than you normally have access to, and so on.

The danger in perceiving that you are doing "it" to another person lies in the burdensome, inflated sense of responsibility that is attached to such a perception.

The individual "receiving" is also acknowledging their ownership and connection with sources of healing energy. The healer is simply acting as a conduit, as a jumper cable connecting and igniting shared energies.

The following exercise will begin to give you an appreciation of your capacity to lend support to a healing process.

Exercise 76 — Healing Experience

1. Let the person who wishes to receive lie on the floor or on a waist-high table. Stand above them. You may want to kneel if they are lying on the floor.
2. Relax yourself and open your heart. (Refer to Exercise 74.)
3. Once you begin to feel warmth, tingling or a surge of energy in your chest, move the energy up to your neck and down your shoulders and arms into your hands.
4. Continue to do this until your hands feel very warm or hot.
5. Now place your hands on or above the area of pain or discomfort and send the energy in your hands to the afflicted area. If the distress is emotional, place your hands on or over the heart.
   a. Let your intuition be your guide as to whether or not you should physically touch the body.
   b. An alternative is to place one hand on your own heart and another on the area of distress.
6. Imagine that the healing energy moves deeply into the body.
   a. You may discover a loss of definition between yourself and the person you are sending energy to. It may be perceived as a sense of having become "one body." Allow yourself to surrender to the sensation.

b. If you become frightened, allow the fear to be felt. It won't harm the other person or you. Conceive of it as simply another emotional block rising to the surface; breathe deeply and allow it to dissolve in the energy flow.

7. You may wish to verbally share images or impressions perceived by each of you during the process, although it is usually preferable to do this at the end of the experience. Feel free to say little or nothing if silence seems most appropriate.

8. Sometimes receiving love and care in this way touches the receiver emotionally and they begin to cry or laugh. This release may be an important part of the healing process. Support this release by staying close or touching an arm. Quietly suggest the advisability of deep slow breathing in regaining equilibrium.

Unconditional loving energy can be sent at any time to anyone with beneficial effects. It follows that the more often you focus on opening your heart, the greater your experience of well-being.

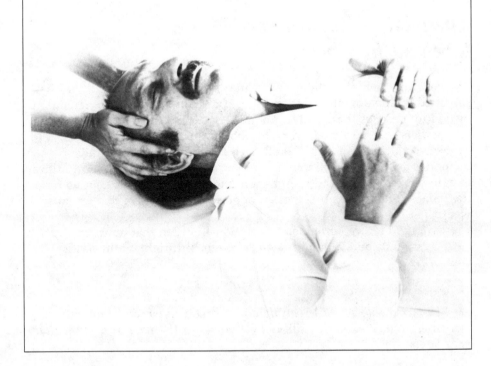

The relationship between conflict and unconditional love

Conflict can be an opportunity to deepen love, as well as the occasion for the power struggle it so often becomes.

Conflict evokes our most protected and hidden emotions, including rage, abandon, fear and hurt. There is a moment of choice sparked by conflict, a moment when we can either withdraw and protect ourselves from the awareness of these emotions or learn about ourselves from them. "Protective" choices include withdrawal, punishment and blame. Learning that leads to enhanced well-being takes place when attention is turned inward to the source of our vulnerability in the midst of conflict. When we do this, our capacity for unconditional love is extended. Energy formerly tied up in protective systems is released and can be used to create a more satisfying life. *The more awareness we permit ourselves to have about our vulnerability, the more loving, energetic and powerful we become.*

The relationship between love and forgiveness

For many, some conflicts seem unresolvable. Memories from the past saturated with pain, anger, bitterness and resentment preoccupy attention or lead to lifestyles that revolve around the need to erase hurtful memories. Addicts drawn to food, work, alcohol or drugs are caught in this protective pattern—victims of their desire to forget. When painful memories and the determination to forget are recognized as opportunities to gain understanding and compassion, then that which has kept us from the fullness of our lives becomes an opportunity to forgive that extends well-being.

By forgiving, we surrender an emotional burden that limits spiritual awareness, and come around full circle to our birthright, enthusiastic well-being.

The following exercise can help you become aware of thoughts or memories connected with pain and bitterness in the past or present that may be limiting.

Exercise 77 — Forgiving

1. Deeply relax yourself.
2. Visualize writing the word "forgiveness" in the sky. Now attach strings to this image. Make the experience as vivid as possible. Remember you need not actually "see" in order to have the experience.
3. Now pose the question, "Who or what do I need to forgive?" and allow whatever happens to happen.
4. Ask the person or situation you are connecting to for clarity and understanding.
5. If you are able, forgive them. If not, don't force yourself, but simply be aware of the resentment you are holding and its consequences in your life.

Conclusion

One of the most amazing characteristics of spiritual awareness is that it brings with it an intensified self-valuing and mental clarity. Life takes on new purpose and possibility as limiting physical, mental, emotional and social boundaries disappear. Unconditional love is a living meditation that dissolves old patterns and constrictions while inspiring new physical, mental, emotional and social development, all of which leads to enthusiastic well-being.

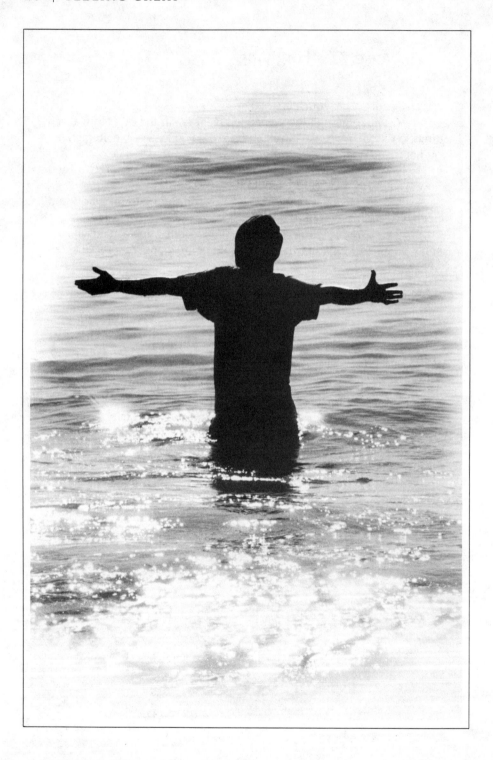

Notes to Chapter VI

[1]The material in this chapter developed out of my work with Dr. B. Joy (See *Joy's Way*). During the last three years I have included the material presented here in my classes and work with private clients and patients at the Center. See also R. Dass, *The Only Dance There Is*; K. von Durckheim, *Daily Life as Spiritual Exercise*; R. DeRopp, *The Master Game: Pathways to Higher Consciousness Beyond the Drug Experience*; Swami Prabhavananda, *The Song of God: Bhagavad-Gita*; B. Rajneesh, *Meditation: The Art of Ecstasy*; A. Watts, *Beyond Theology* and *The Joyous Cosmology*.

[2]See R. DeRopp, *The Master Game: Pathways to Higher Consciousness Beyond the Drug Experience* and B. Payne, *Getting There Without Drugs*.

[3]I was first introduced to energy work by Dr. B. Joy (see *Joy's Way*). Later I studied with Dr. Harold Stone and now routinely work with energy in my private practice and with patients at the Center for the Healing Arts. Personal experience has convinced me that psychological and physical healing is facilitated by the process of recognizing and extending this subtler energy.

[4]This exercise is one used by Dr. Stone in introducing energy work to people unfamiliar with it.

[5]See B. Gunther, *Energy Ecstasy*.

[6]For more help with relaxed gazing, turn to the section on "Soft Eyes" in the Appendix to G. Leonard, *The Silent Pulse*.

[7]Cf. Dr. B. Joy's work (see *Joy's Way*).

[8]This conclusion is drawn from my personal experience over the last three years working with patients and students.

[9]The conclusions drawn in this section and the next section are based on my work at the Center for the Healing Arts.

Postlude:
Illness as Teacher

The following impressions and observations are based on the work I've done with seriously ill people at the Center for the Healing Arts in Los Angeles.[1] The Center treats people with catastrophic diseases, such as cancer, from a holistic perspective. This means that the sources of well-being described and explored in this book are looked to in an attempt to understand the disequilibrium that led to illness. Physical, mental, emotional and spiritual needs are considered as possible causal and contributing factors in the disease process.[2]

All participants at the Center are under medical supervision. The holistic principles complementing traditional medical care might be summarized as follows:

1. Health is no less than ecstatic well-being. It is not simply a disease- or distress-free state. In life, something must replace that which has been taken away. Permanent cure thus has as much to do with exploring and choosing "health" as it does with mending or removing illness.

2. Distress and illness can be viewed as the body's attempt to right imbalance and bring about equilibrium. Illness from this perspective becomes a teacher or guide to health. In this context, among the first questions to ask, after severe symptoms such as bleeding have been stopped are:

    a. What is this illness saying to me?

    b. What am I missing in life?

    c. What am I refusing to see or do?

These questions and others like them can, of course, be worked with in any number of ways suggested in this book, including guide meditation, voice dialogue, personal journal and dreams.

3. We are active participants in the processes that result in distress and illness, as well as in regaining health and well-being. And, like well-being, the choice depends on awareness. Without awareness, respon-

sible choice is inhibited. Blaming ourselves for the things we "should have done or known" is counterproductive to healing or well-being. The point is not to waste energy regretting the past, but to use the energy to explore and extend awareness in the present.

4. Taking responsibility for healing ourselves *does not mean refusing help*. Active participation includes understanding when we need assistance and having the capacity to reach out appropriately for it. Western medical science has much to offer a responsible and informed person. When we are open to receiving help, one path is as worth exploring as another. Eventually we will select the course of action that seems most promising and apply ourselves to it.

5. Blame and recrimination represent as great a danger to health as does drinking contaminated water. Punishment, criticism and faultfinding close our hearts and produce stress. Energy invested in lamenting and regretting the behavior of ourselves or others is energy no longer available for purposes of gaining self-awareness and enhancing the quality of life.

6. Denial of that which we need or very much want is stressful and unhealthy for many people. Further, when needs are connected with the approval of others, fear, resentment and blame are often the consequences. The avoidance of conflict can lead to distress and illness. Conflict, which results from the attachment to differing points of view, is an inescapable part of civilized life. Within the context of a desire to understand rather than blame, conflict seeds awareness and well-being by drawing attention to these attachments.

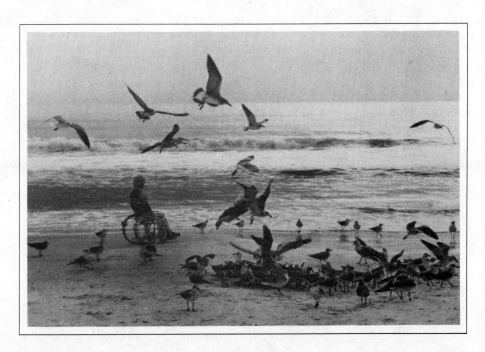

7. Illness and death can free people from a burdensome sense of responsibility that interferes with the pursuit of extended awareness and well-being. Responsibility is not sacrifice, but rather response-ability— the capacity to respond appropriately to other people and life in general. That which is appropriate will enhance the well-being of all.

8. Consciousness of impending death can greatly enhance the quality of life. When people use serious illness as an opportunity to explore the choices they have made, along with new possibilities, the dying process can include well-being.

9. Service supports a healing process. Caring for others, or giving to others in ways that make us feel good, lends meaning and purpose to life. A common cause of deep stress is the belief that we have no effect on life. Service rights this imbalance.

10. Playfulness, fun and laughter are tremendously facilitating to the healing process. The capacity to laugh with others and at oneself is a key to relaxing the fear and judgments that can stress us so.

Notes to Postlude

[1] I've been a member of the senior staff working in the research clinic with seriously ill individuals and illness groups in the capacity of a psychotherapist and holistic guide.

[2] The Center community is one that permits an intensive ongoing relationship between staff and patients. The material summarized here not only draws upon my experience co-leading transformational groups at the Center but reflects what I have learned by knowing individual patients personally.

Bibliography

Alexander, F. M. *The Resurrection of the Body.* New York: University Books, 1969.

Assagioli, R. *The Act of Will.* New York: Viking Press, 1973.

Barlow, W. *The Alexander Technique.* New York: Alfred A. Knopf, 1973.

Boston Women's Health Book Collective. *Our Bodies, Ourselves.* New York: Simon and Schuster, 1971.

Brain/Mind Bulletin, published twice a month and edited by Marilyn Ferguson. Reports on current developments in brain research and consciousness. Available from Interface Press, P.O. Box 42211, Los Angeles, California, 90042.

Brown, B. *New Mind, New Body.* New York: Harper and Row, 1974.

Calder, N. *The Mind of Man.* New York: Viking Compass, 1970.

Cooper, K. H. *The New Aerobics.* New York: M. Evans, 1970.

Cousins, N. *Anatomy of an Illness As Perceived by the Patient: Reflections on Healing and Regeneration.* New York: W. W. Norton, 1979.

Dass, R. *Journey of Awakening: A Meditator's Guidebook.* New York: Bantam Books, 1978.

Dass, R. *The Only Dance There Is.* Garden City, New York: Anchor, 1974.

Dentan, R. K. *The Semai: A Non-violent People of Malaya.* New York: Holt, Rinehart and Winston, 1968.

DeRopp, R. *The Master Game: Pathways to Higher Consciousness Beyond the Drug Experience.* New York: Delacorte, 1968.

Durckheim, K. von. *Daily Life as Spiritual Exercise: The Way of Transformation.* New York: Perennial Library, 1972.

Einstein, A. *The Meaning of Relativity.* Princeton: Princeton University Press, 1971.

Fay, M. *The Dream Guide.* Los Angeles: Center for the Healing Arts, 1978.

Feldenkrais, M. *Awareness Through Movement.* New York: Harper and Row, 1972.

Ferguson, M. *The Brain Revolution.* New York: Bantam Books, 1975.

Friedman, M., and Rosenman, R. H. *Type A Behavior and Your Heart.* New York: Alfred A. Knopf, 1974.

Fromm, E. *The Art of Loving.* New York: Harper and Row, 1956.

Geba, B. *Breathe Away Your Tension.* New York: Random House and Berkeley: The Bookworks, 1973.

Gunther, B. *Energy Ecstasy.* Los Angeles: The Guild of Tutors Press, 1978.

Herrigel, E. *Zen.* Tr. by R. F. C. Hull. New York: McGraw-Hill, 1964.

Herrigel, E. *Zen in the Art of Archery.* Tr. by R. F. C. Hull. New York: Vintage Books, 1971.

Hittleman, R. *Introduction to Yoga.* New York: Bantam Books, 1969.

Iyengar, B. K. S. *Light on Yoga.* New York: Schocken Books, 1973.

Joy, W. B. *Joy's Way.* Los Angeles: J. P. Tarcher, 1979.

Jung, C. G. *Memories, Dreams, Reflections.* Tr. by Richard Winston and Clara Winston. New York: Pantheon, 1963.

Katz, J. *Dreams Are Your Truest Friends.* New York: Pocket Books, 1976.

Keys, L. *Toning.* Marina del Ray, California: DeVorss, 1973.

Leonard, G. *The Silent Pulse.* New York: E. P. Dutton, 1978.

Lindemann, H. *Relieve Tension the Autogenic Way.* Tr. by Konrad Keller. New York: P. H. Wyden, 1973.

McKim, R. H. *Experiences in Visual Thinking.* Monterey, California: Brooks/Cole, 1972.

Masters, R., and Houston, J. *Mind Games.* New York: Viking Press, 1972.

Nin, A. *The Diary of Anais Nin, 1931–1934.* New York: Harcourt, Brace and World, 1966.

Paul, M., and Paul, J. *Free to Love.* Los Angeles: J. P. Tarcher, 1975.

Payne, B. *Getting There Without Drugs.* New York: Viking Press, 1973.

Pearce, J. C. *The Crack in the Cosmic Egg*. New York: Pocket Books, 1973.

Pendleton, B., and Mehling, B. *Relax! with Self-Therap/Ease*. Calabasas, California: California Publications, 1976.

Perls, F. *Gestalt Therapy Verbatim*. Lafayette, California: Real People Press, 1969.

Perls, F. *In and Out the Garbage Pail*. Lafayette, California: Real People Press, 1969.

Pirsig, R. *Zen and the Art of Motorcycle Maintenance*. New York: Bantam Books, 1976.

Prabhavananda, Swami, and Isherwood, C., tr. *The Song of God: Bhagavad-Gita*. New York: New American Library, 1951.

Progoff, I. *At a Journal Workshop: The Basic Text and Guide for Using the Intensive Journal*. New York: Dialogue House Library, 1975.

Rajneesh, B. *Meditation: The Art of Ecstasy*. New York: Harper Colophon, 1976.

Rogers, C. R. *On Becoming a Person*. Boston: Houghton Mifflin, 1961.

Rogers, C. R., and Stevens, B. *Person to Person*. New York: Pocket Books, 1971.

Rosenberg, J. *Total Orgasm*. New York: Random House and Berkeley: The Bookworks, 1973.

Rush, A. K. *Getting Clear*. New York: Random House and Berkeley: The Bookworks, 1973.

Samples, B. *The Metaphoric Mind: A Celebration of Creative Consciousness*. Reading, Massachusetts, Addison-Wesley, 1976.

Satir, V. *Peoplemaking*. Palo Alto, California: Science and Behavior Books, 1972.

Schoop, T., and Mitchell, P. *Won't You Join the Dance?* Palo Alto, California: Mayfield Publishing Co., 1974.

Selye, H. *The Stress of Life*. Rev. ed. New York: McGraw-Hill, 1976.

Selye, H. *Stress Without Distress*. New York: J. P. Lippincott, 1974.

Simonton, O. C., and Simonton, S. S. "Belief Systems and Management of the Emotional Aspects of Malignancy." *Journal of Transpersonal Psychology*, 1975, pp. 29–47.

Smith, A. *Powers of Mind*. New York: Ballantine, 1976.

Stevens, B. *Don't Push the River*. Moab, Utah: Real People Press, 1970.

Stevens, J. *Awareness: Exploring, Experimenting, Experiencing*. New York: Bantam Books, 1973.

Stone, H., and Winkelman, S. "Voice Dialogue: A Tool for Transformation." Copies available at the Center for the Healing Arts, West Los Angeles.

Toben, B., and Sarfatti, J. *Space-Time and Beyond*. New York: E. P. Dutton, 1975.

Watts, A. *Beyond Theology: The Art of Godmanship*. New York: Vintage Books, 1973.

Watts, A. *The Joyous Cosmology*. New York: Vintage Books, 1970.